the Abs Diet

6-Minute Meals for 6-Pack Abs

the Abs Diet

6-Minute Meals for 6-Pack Abs

DAVID ZINCZENKO, Editor-in-Chief of **Men'sHealth**

WITH TED SPIKER

RODALE

Some portions of this book have appeared previously in *Men's Health* magazine.

Book design by Christopher Rhoads

Library of Congress Cataloging-in-Publication Data

Zinczenko, David.
   The abs diet 6-minute meals for 6-pack abs / David Zinczenko ; with Ted Spiker.
      p.   cm.
   Includes index.
   ISBN-13: 978–1–59486–546–6 (hardcover)
   ISBN-10: 1–59486–546–9 (hardcover)
   1. Reducing diets. 2. Reducing diets—Recipes. 3. Nutrition. 4. Abdomen—Muscles.
 I. Spiker, Ted. II. Title.
   RM222.2.Z557 2006
   613.2'5 dc22   2006008648

Distributed to the trade by Holtzbrinck Publishers

    6 8 10 9 7 5   hardcover

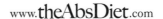

To all the men and women struggling to stay fit and healthy in our hectic, harried world. It's time to take control of our food supply and stop swallowing what the junk merchants are cooking up.

Contents

Acknowledgments

Seeing the Abs Diet series come to fruition has been one of the great pleasures of my life. Seeing it make a real impact on the lives of tens of thousands of Americans has been one of the great rewards. For all of it, I have to thank a number of extraordinarily talented, hardworking, and dedicated people who continue to support, encourage, and inspire me. In particular:

Steve Murphy, whose courage and commitment to editorial quality have made Rodale Inc. the best publishing company in the world to work for.

The Rodale family, without whom none of this would be possible.

Ben Roter, whom I want to be when I grow up.

Ted Spiker, the world's best coauthor.

Steve Perrine, who works his creative magic day in and day out.

The entire *Men's Health* editorial staff, the smartest and hardest-working group of writers, editors, researchers, designers, and photo directors in the industry.

A big shout-out to Phillip Rhodes, Rob Gerth, Kathryn C. LeSage, Chris Krogermeier, Chris Rhoads, Hope Clarke, Kathleen Hanuschak, Keith Biery, Brenda Miller, and everyone else who worked so hard and so fast to publish this book.

My brother, Eric, whose relentless teasing shamed me into taking better care of myself. (Dude, you're sooo dead. . . .)

My mother, Janice, who raised two of us nearly single-handedly. Your strength and kindness guide my every action.

My dad, Bohdan, who left this world way too early. I wish you were still here.

My uncle, Denny Stanz, the picture of youthfulness.

My stepmother, Mickey, ditto.

Elaine Kaufman, who still lets me order off the menu.

And special thanks to: Dan Abrams, Jeff Anthony, Jeff Beacher (get on the plan!), Matt Bean, Mary Ann Bekkedahl, Tami Booth Corwin, Mark Bricklin, Michael Bruno, Marianne Butler, Adam Campbell, Jeff Csatari, Jack Essig, Kimberly Guilfoyle, Jon Hammond and Karen Mazzotta, Joe Heroun, Erin Hobday, Samantha Irwin, George Karabotsos, Charlene Lutz, MM and RP!, Vincent Maggio, Paul McGinley, Patrick McMullan, Peter Moore, Jeff Morgan, Paige Nelson, Sarah Peters, John Phelan, Bill Phillips, Richard and Sessa, Scott Quill, Eric Sacks, David Schipper, Zachary Schisgal, Leslie Schneider, Larry Shire, Joyce Shirer, Bill Stanton, Bill Stump, John Tayman, and Pat and Steve Toomey. Thanks for all the rock-solid advice. You guys rule.

Introduction

GIVE ME 6 MINUTES FOR YOUR MEALS, AND I'LL GIVE YOU A 6-PACK FOR LIFE

A **LOT CAN HAPPEN IN 6 MINUTES.**
Six minutes is all the time it takes for a Kenyan marathoner to run more than a mile and for a rocket headed to Pluto to cover nearly 5,000 miles. Six minutes is the approximate length of some of our careers (think any first-round *Apprentice* casualty) and some of our marriages ("Welcome back to Las Vegas, Ms. Spears!"). Six minutes is enough time to make or break a job interview, have unforgettable sex, or listen to all of Quiet Riot's greatest hits.

And in 6 minutes, you can find your 6-pack of abs.

ABS FACT

2.5

Number of times more likely an obese person is to die in a car crash, compared with a thin person

—*Accident Analysis and Prevention*

Not with a CAT scan, or an endoscope, or a self-powered liposuction vacuum, but with an intelligent, well-balanced, great-tasting, and (most of all) easy eating plan. Not a fad diet. Not three meals a day of grapefruit juice and tofu dogs. And no weird vacuum-sealed meals that have to be special-delivered to your home by the food police. Just sensible food that's fast and easy—and that doesn't get pushed through the window of your car by a guy in a paper hat.

But in today's society, eating sensibly is a lot harder than it might seem. We live in a fast-paced world, one dominated by "convenience" food, "fast" food, "ready-to-eat" food. Even if you never step foot in a Burger Sting or Taco Hell, even if you eat every meal sitting at your own kitchen table—or, if you're a bachelor, standing over your kitchen sink—the majority of the food you eat probably comes out of a box, a bag, or a can. And the price for all that convenience is being rung up every day—on your waistline.

Remember the adage about war: An army travels on its stomach. If you want to win the battle against your belly, you need to control your food. You need to know exactly what's going into your body and exactly what it's doing *to* your body.

Abs, after all, aren't made in the gym—they're made in the kitchen. What you put into your mouth is far more important than what you put into your work-out. For example, in a meta-analysis of 33 clinical trials, Brazilian researchers determined that diet controls about 75 percent of weight loss. Of course, that doesn't mean exercise isn't an important part of the fat-burning formula. But if you want the fastest results, working out isn't enough; a smart eating plan is the foundation of an effective gut-busting program. And that's what this book is all about.

The Amazing Benefits of the Abs Diet

WHEN I DEVELOPED the Abs Diet in 2004, I had one mission: I wanted to give people their best bodies and highest levels of health without taking up all of their time. To do that, I developed the Abs Diet Powerfoods—12 classes of food that are so body- and palate-friendly (and easy to remember) that they can change your body—and your life—forever. They do things like boost your metabolism, lower your cholesterol, decrease your hunger, raise your standing at the doctor's office, and increase the likelihood that you'll need to buy smaller pants. Best of all, they help you change your body so that you're burning more fat, adding more lean muscle, and losing the weight that you want. Just imagine your life with . . .

▶ **A leaner, fitter body.** The ultimate goal of the Abs Diet—and of the meals you'll find in these pages—is to reset your body's metabolism. You do that by building lean, mean, fat-burning muscle through exercise and through eating the right foods, like the meals described within. In fact, between 60 and 80 percent of the calories you burn in any given day aren't burned by jogging or biking or racing to catch your flight after getting stopped and felt up by airport security (again). They're burned simply in order to keep your body tissue alive and functioning. And much of that calorie burn goes to supporting your muscles. Add a few pounds of muscle, and your body has no choice but to burn away fat to support that muscle. In other words, you're not just going to lose weight, you're going to change your physique entirely—and for good!

▶ **Better sex.** Sure, abs will make you more appealing to the opposite sex (heads up, guys—in one survey, 32 percent of women said abs were the muscles that most made them melt, with biceps a distant second at 17 percent). But abs will also get your mojo working like never before. See, the same plaque that forms in your arteries and leads you toward heart disease also gums up the works in your nether regions. For men, that means softer erections (overweight men are 50 percent more likely to suffer erectile dysfunction); for women, it means less lubrication and a diminished sexual response. The Abs Diet counteracts these effects, helping maintain and maximize your sexual machinery.

▶ **A longer, healthier future.** In a recent Canadian study of more than 8,000 people, researchers found that over 13 years, those with the weakest abdominal muscles had a death rate twice as high as those with the strongest midsections. In an American study of more than 22,000 men, those with waists larger than 36.8 inches had significantly elevated risk of heart attack. (And the real scary part? That's actually

2 inches *smaller* than the waist of the average American male!) Would you rather be out chasing a thrill or sitting at home writing your will? I thought so. . . .

▶ **Less stress, greater happiness, and more life satisfaction.** Consider this: Overweight people are more likely to suffer from everything from knee pain to hip pain to carpal tunnel syndrome. They're 20 percent more likely to have asthma; 14 percent more likely to develop osteoarthritis; 70 percent more likely to develop high blood pressure. Overweight people make an average of $3,000 less per year and are 14 percent less attractive to the opposite sex. Losing weight and finding your abs isn't just about looking better—it's about feeling better and living better, too!

ABS FACT

8.6

Average percentage by which your level of body fat could increase if you quit exercising for 8 months

—*University of North Carolina*

And that brings us to *The Abs Diet 6-Minute Meals for 6-Pack Abs.* In order to help you see all of those promises come true, I decided to apply the principles of the Abs Diet to create a batch of easy-to-make meals that are just as fast, convenient, and delicious as anything the Colonel or Aunt Jemima or that Redenbacher guy can cook up.

See, whether you're talking about a lover, a get-rich scheme, or a meal, "cheap, fast, and easy" almost always means one thing: trouble. In my job as editor-in-chief of *Men's Health* magazine, I hear about weight-loss successes—

and failures—every day. I read studies about what works for people and what doesn't, and I ingest nutritional information the way Joe Rogan's guests ingest blended worms. And what I've learned from all of my research on the modern diet is that, as Cat Stevens might say, "A lot of nice things turn bad out there."

Modern convenience foods are laced with fat-promoting ingredients like trans fats and high-fructose corn syrup (HFCS). These ingredients not only make us fat, they make us want to eat more—and get even fatter. And we go right along, playing into the hands of food manufacturers who want nothing more than to make us buy—and eat—more of their food. It's a vicious cycle: We eat food that doesn't satisfy us, so we crave more, and that doesn't satisfy us either, and so we eat even more. You'll read more about these and other dietary evils—and why you need to take control of your food in order to avoid them—in an upcoming chapter.

How to Fight Back—And Fight Fat!

IT MAY SEEM obvious, but the key to getting a handle on your weight is to get a handle on what's going into your body. That means weaning yourself off convenience food without sacrificing the convenience. Let's face it: Life is fast-paced and clamorous. It's easy to swing by the drive-thru, or slide a few dollars into the vending machine, or grab whatever's in the pantry and start shoveling it into your maw. The only way to control what you eat is to make your own meals. And the only way you're going to take the time to make your own meals consistently

ABS FACT

150,000

Gallons of fat, on average, sucked out of people and subsequently discarded by plastic surgeons each year

—*International Fat Applied Technology Society*

is if those meals are simple to whip up and the most delightful thing to happen to your mouth since your first under-the-bleachers kiss.

And making fast, delicious meals is what this book will empower you to do.

Since the *New York Times* bestseller *The Abs Diet* came out, I've seen thousands of people lose their guts, regain their health, and change their bodies, and I know the reason why the Abs Diet works so well.

It's because the food guidelines are easy to remember. It's because the Abs Diet is easy, is nutritious, and gives you the things we all crave, whether at work, in the bedroom, or in the kitchen: variety and flexibility. In fact, one recent Tufts University study showed that the less restrictive a diet plan, the better your chance of long-term weight loss.

All of the quick and easy meals in this book are based on the principles of the Abs Diet and the Abs Diet Powerfoods—the 12 groups of healthy proteins, healthy fats, and healthy carbohydrates that will help you lose weight and stay full all day. Here's a quick introduction to the not-so-dirty dozen:

THE ABS DIET POWER 12

Almonds and other nuts

Beans and legumes

Spinach and other green vegetables

Dairy (fat-free or low-fat milk, yogurt, cheese)

Instant oatmeal (unsweetened, unflavored)

Eggs

Turkey and other lean meats

Peanut butter

Olive oil

Whole grain breads and cereals

Extra-protein (whey) powder

Raspberries and other berries

Remember the Abs Diet Power 12, and you'll be armed with the information you need to eat right whether you're at home, in the office, or on the road; whether you're living in your dream home or in a dorm, in the barracks or at Mom's house. Build your meals around these foods, and you'll have taken the first big step toward achieving your abdominal goals.

ABS FACT

34

Percentage increase in an overweight person's overall likelihood of developing cancer

—*American Journal of Epidemiology*

Good Gosh, Let's Eat Already!

MOST OF US equate diet with deprivation—the idea being that if you eat less, you'll weigh less. But the Abs Diet isn't about making you feel more deprived than a middle child. It's about constantly fueling your body with Powerfoods. The Abs Diet isn't about eating less, having less, being less. It's about eating, having, and being MORE.

▶ Most diets want you to eat less food. I want you to eat more.

▶ Most diets want you to eat less often. I want you to eat more often.

▶ Most diets restrict you by calories, or grams, or "zones." And quite frankly, I just don't have time to worry about all that nonsense—do you?

I'll never tell you that you have to eat Food X at Time Y and that you better wash it down with Drink Z. I'll give you the tools to make decisions about what and when you eat and dozens and dozens of quick and easy meals to whip up whenever you want a bite. But *you're* the one who's in charge of this eating plan. To me, that's an important part of making the switch from feeling like you're on a diet to actually adopting a healthier eating approach every day.

And just look at what you'll get once you make that switch:

▶ **More meals.** If you go on a diet that emphasizes restriction and denial, you're simply teaching your body to store fat. That's right: When you don't eat, you store fat. That's because your body senses you're in starvation mode, so it makes its own fat emergency kit—storing fat to use for energy

ABS FACT

23.1

Percentage of Americans who consume five or more servings of fruits and vegetables per day

—*Centers for Disease Control and Prevention*

in case the lean times continue. A recent study in the *American Journal of Preventive Medicine* found that about 60 percent of Americans who try to lose weight do so by restricting their calorie intake, with roughly one in 10 skipping meals in a desperate attempt to strip off the pounds. But study after study has shown that yo-yo dieting is one of the best ways to ensure your belly will get bigger.

The truth is that in order to burn fat, you have to eat more often—to the tune of six meals a day. That frequent intake of calories reminds your body that it has the energy it needs to keep you moving and that it can afford to dump that unsightly fat it's been carrying around. Eating at a pace of once every couple of hours also keeps you full, so that you're never experiencing the huge hunger pangs that lead to ravenous snacking.

▶ **More nutrition.** When you base your meals on the Abs Diet Power 12, you automatically boost the nutritional quality of your diet. You'll get more vitamins, minerals, and fiber (crucial for preventing diseases like cancer and heart disease); more protein and calcium (both of which help you turn useless flab into lean, mean muscle); and more healthy fats like monounsaturated fats and omega-3s (which help keep your arteries clear and slash your risk of heart attack and stroke).

▶ **More muscle.** We used to equate muscle mass with bodybuilders, football players, and Eastern Bloc female swim teams. It's time we started associating muscle mass with one more thing: weight loss. For every pound of muscle you add, your body burns up to 50 extra calories of fat a day, just to maintain that muscle.

Now, hold on—I know what you're thinking, and no, this plan won't turn you into the next Iron Mike Tyson. No one will confuse you with the Incredible Hulk or ask you to join the WWF. We're talking about very moderate gains: Add just 6 pounds of muscle (about the size of a man's bicep) to your entire physique, and you'll be burning up to an extra 300 calories a day. That's 300 calories you melt away every single day just by sleeping, or driving, or surfing the Web. Of course, you'll build much of that muscle with exercise (see pages 232 through 239, as well as my book *The Abs Diet Get Fit, Stay Fit Plan* for specifics). But you'll also build it by eating foods—specifically ones high in protein— that have been shown to help add fat-burning muscle.

The best part about this approach to eating is that you can power your physical machine with the highest-quality fuel and end up with the healthy and lean body that you want—simply by using these 6-minute meals.

Make them, eat them, and watch your belly change from fat to flat.

Come to think of it, it all really does come down to one simple equation:

12 ABS DIET POWERFOODS + 6 MINUTES = YOUR 6-PACK ABS

THE ABS DIET NUTRITION CHEAT SHEET

SUBJECT	GUIDELINE
Number of meals	Six a day, spaced relatively evenly throughout the day. Eat snacks 2 hours before larger meals.
The **ABS DIET POWER 12**	Base most of your meals on these 12 groups of foods. Every meal should have at least two foods from the list.

Almonds and other nuts
Beans and legumes
Spinach and other green vegetables

Dairy (fat-free or low-fat milk, yogurt, cheese)
Instant oatmeal (unsweetened, unflavored)
Eggs
Turkey and other lean meats

Peanut butter
Olive oil
Whole grain breads and cereals
Extra-protein (whey) powder
Raspberries and other berries

SUBJECT	GUIDELINE
Portion size	While it's always important to consider the amounts of food you eat, the Abs Diet, in a way, acts to self-regulate your portions. The high-fiber, high-protein foods will fill you up and help control your hunger. If you space out your meals with just a few hours between them and make the Abs Diet Power 12 foods the majority of your diet, your body will tell you when it's time to eat—and when it's time to stop.
Secret weapons	Each of the Abs Diet Power 12 has been chosen in part for its stealthy, healthy secret weapons—the nutrients that will help power up your natural fat burners, protect you from illness and injury, and keep you lean and fit for life!
Nutritional allies	Protein, monounsaturated and polyunsaturated fats, fiber, calcium
Nutritional enemies	Refined carbohydrates (or carbs with a high glycemic index), saturated fats, trans fats, high-fructose corn syrup
Alcohol	Limit yourself to two or three drinks per week, to maximize the benefits of the Abs Diet plan.
Ultimate Powerfood	Smoothies. The calcium and protein in milk, yogurt, whey powder, and peanut butter, combined with the fiber in oatmeal and fruit, make them one of the more filling and easy options. Drink them regularly.
Cheating	One meal a week, eat anything you want.

Chapter I

THE SUPERHEROES OF 6-PACK

The Nutrients That Will Help You Find Your Abs— And the Villains That Plot Against You

EVEN IF YOU SPEND ABOUT as much time with comic books as Ron Howard spends with hair gel, you know the story line of every superhero tale—whether it involves Superman, Underdog, or the Incredibles. It's hero vs. villain, good vs. evil, bat wings vs. unsolvable riddles. At stake: a city, a woman, the world, box-office rankings.

Inside your body, the same kinds of battles take place with the same kinds of heroes and villains (minus the underwear worn *over* the tights). At stake: your body.

See, food has the power to either save your body or destroy it, and by choosing what you eat, you determine the ultimate nutritional fate: whether the good powers prevail and the bad ones are vanquished.

The Villains: The Flabtastic Four

The Villain: The Sweet Masquerader
Given Name: High-Fructose Corn Syrup (HFCS)

Primary Evil Powers: Identity theft; inflicts intense hunger pains.
Nutritional Crimes: This artificial sweetener that masquerades as sugar is twice as sinister as the sucrose it impersonates. Bearing primary responsibility for the collective weight gain in our society, the Sweet Masquerader hypnotizes eaters into thinking they're always hungry. Here's how this little bugger was born: About 30 years ago, food manufacturers figured out that they could make sodas, cereals, yogurts, and some 40,000 other manufactured foods taste sweeter—for a lot less money than with simple sugar. They did it by developing HFCS (which is derived from corn). Sounds fine in theory, but here's the

ABS FACT

72 Percentage of Americans who don't check nutrition labels or content before buying food

problem: When you eat any type of carbohydrate (like bread or fruit), your body releases insulin to regulate your body weight, pushing those carb calories into your muscles to be used as energy or storing them for later. Then it suppresses

FOODS HIGH IN HFCS	REPLACE WITH
Regular soft drinks	Unsweetened sparkling water
Commercial candy (jelly beans and others)	Chocolate candy (check the label, though—some chocolate candy bars may use HFCS as an ingredient)
Apple juice (typically about 60% fructose)	Unrefined 100% apple juice, grape juice, orange juice, or (here's a shocker) whole fruit
Pancake syrup	Real maple syrup
Popsicles	Frozen-fruit bars (always check the label; some brands may have added HFCS)
Frozen yogurt	Fat-free or low-fat ice cream
Fruit-flavored yogurt	Artificially sweetened or sugar-sweetened fat-free or low-fat yogurt
Ketchup	Mustard
Highly sweetened cereals	Sugar-free or low-sugar cereals
Pasta sauce (especially Ragu)	Sugar-free pasta sauce
Canned soup	Organic, all-natural, or sugar-free soups (check the label—an HFCS-free soup won't list any sugar)

ABS FACT

5 Number of pounds the average 180-pound man gains during the first 2 years of marriage. What's worse: 44 percent of women found the excess pounds to "detrimentally affect the relationship."

your appetite. Those carbs are the signal for you to stop filling your tank. But the Sweet Masquerader doesn't stimulate insulin, so your body doesn't register it the way it registers simple white sugar. (That's why you can drink a few Big Gulps and never really feel full.) So what are you left with? You eat the HFCS-containing foods that are high in calories, but, like a band that stops after one set, those foods leave you wanting more. So you eat more foods with HFCS, stockpiling those calories like they're savings bonds, and the cycle of eating—and storing fat—continues.

Attack Plan: Today, you can find HFCS in things like ketchup, pasta sauce, and crackers—it's everywhere. Now, you don't need to eliminate it completely (though that's the ideal), but you do need to treat it like a manipulative ex and find ways to kick it out of your life. If HFCS is listed first or second on an ingredients list, see how many grams of "sugars" (HFCS is lumped in that category) the food product contains. If there's just a gram or two, that's okay. But if a food has 8 or more grams of sugars and HFCS is prominent on the list of ingredients, ditch that grub.

The Villain: The Blob
Given Name: Trans Fat

Primary Evil Powers: Turns fat in foods into fat on your belly.

Nutritional Crimes: "Trans fats" may sound like the name of a cross-dressing pool hustler, but the reality is even more bizarre. Artificially made fats, trans fats are like wigs in shower drains—mammoth cloggers. They gunk up the works by increasing the amount of bad cholesterol in your body. (Trans fats have been linked to an increased risk of heart disease and diabetes.) You can understand why when you realize how they're made. Trans fats are created by combining vegetable oil (a liquid) with hydrogen to create partially hydrogenated oil, or trans fatty acids. Once infused with the hydrogen, the liquid vegetable oil turns into a solid at room temperature. And the food industry loves trans fats, because they are cheap and seem to stick around forever. Plus, you can add trans fats to all kinds of foods in a way you can't add regular oil (for instance, normal vegetable oil in a cookie recipe would ooze out when the weather gets warm; with trans fats, the treats stay crisp and solid). So now trans fats—like HFCS—get added to chips, fries, muffins, and all sorts of on-the-shelf products. But the real evil is what the Blob does to you on the inside. Remember, these fats are supposed to be liquid but have turned into solid. So instead of melting, like they would in their natural state, inside your body, they try to revert to their waxy, solid makeup—inside your arteries.

Attack Plan: Scan the label and eliminate. Like hotel bars on business trips, little good can come from them. Some tips for total avoidance:

▶ Check ingredients lists for aliases like "hydrogenated" or "partially hydrogenated." The higher these ingredients are on the label, the more trans fats they contain.

▶ Pick high-protein breakfasts like eggs and Canadian bacon over waffles. If you have toast, skip the margarine. Processed bread products and margarine are two of the most common forms in which trans fats find their way into our bodies.

▶ At a restaurant, ask what kind of oil the chef uses. You want to hear olive oil, not shortening (another code name for the Blob).

▶ When eating out, stick to soup or salad and avoid the bread, which can be filled with trans fats.

FOODS CONTAINING TRANS FAT	REPLACE WITH
Spreads: stick margarine, shortening, butter	Almond or natural peanut butter Soft tub margarines (less likely to have trans fats) Land O' Lakes whipped butter (50 percent fewer calories than stick and doesn't contain trans fat) Benecol (a butter and margarine alternative)
Frozen food: pies, pot pies, pizza, waffles, breaded fish sticks	Frozen stir-fry with chicken, beef, or shrimp Grilled salmon Frozen fruit pops Kellogg's Special K fat-free waffles

(continued)

FOODS CONTAINING TRANS FAT	REPLACE WITH
Baked goods and shells: doughnuts, cream-filled cookies, pound cake, muffins, taco shells	Multigrain and whole wheat bread Flour tortillas Angel food or sponge cake Archway fat-free cookies and Pamela's Gourmet cookies
Chips and crackers: potato chips, Wheat Thins, Cheez-It crackers	Pretzels Raisins Walnuts Celery Salsa and natural yellow corn chips Baked chips
Cereals and bars: Kellogg's Cracklin' Oat Bran, Post Selects Great Grains, General Mills Cinnamon Toast Crunch, Quaker Chewy low-fat chocolate chunk granola bars	Whole wheat toast Cereals with nuts (they contain healthy fat) Cheerios Artificially sweetened or sugar-sweetened fat-free or low-fat yogurt Instant oatmeal (unsweetened, unflavored) Post Premium Raisin Bran Eggs and Canadian bacon
Toppings and dip: nondairy creamers, whipped toppings, bean dips, gravy mixes, salad dressings	Fat-free or low-fat milk Oil-and-vinegar dressing Fat-free dips Hummus Olive or sesame oil
Packaged soups: Ramen noodles	Fat-free and reduced-fat canned/packaged soups
Fried fast food: fried chicken and fish, fries	Broiled meat and poultry

The Villain: The Belt Buster
Given Name: Saturated Fats

Primary Evil Powers: Hangs around your midsection, refusing to be burned.
Nutritional Crimes: In a way, saturated fats and trans fats are partners—they're both more likely to be stored than to be burned. While your body likes to burn some kinds of fats as energy (see the Hero on page 24), it would rather save saturated fats around your belly and use them for energy at a future date when food sources are scarce. Problem is, food is never scarce. Since we're lucky enough to live in a time and place where we don't experience famines, droughts, or lack of convenience stores, we don't need that fat, but our bodies still store it. Worse, saturated fats raise cholesterol levels and have also been shown to increase your risk for heart disease and some types of cancer.
Attack Plan: Since saturated fats are usually found in meats and dairy products, you should always choose the leaner forms of protein and the low-fat forms of dairy. Throughout the book, we'll show you ways to find the foods that contain the good stuff (muscle-building protein and fat-fighting calcium) without the bad.

ABS FACT

9.5 Number of pounds gained by those who switch to the night shift. Why? The circadian shift seems to stress the body and promote weight gain.

The Villain: White Fright
Given Name: Refined Carbohydrates

Primary Evil Powers: Nutritional apathy—they don't do a thing.
Nutritional Crimes: Considering that they've gotten more bad press than James Frey, you'd think that we'd have torn all our carbohydrates into a million little pieces by now. But it's a mistake to eliminate all carbs from your diet. You can't survive without carbohydrates, because grains—just like fruits, vegetables, and other food groups—provide crucial energy to feed your brain, muscles, and metabolism, not to mention the fact that they also contain loads of minerals, vitamins, and fiber. The problem really is in refined carbohydrates, such as white sugar, white bread, bagels, white pasta, and waffles. Most of these products are made from grains that have had all their nutrients refined out of them. If you eat the carbs with the grain, the fiber takes up room in your belly and sends you the signal that you're full. But if all the grains are taken out (as is the case with refined carbs like white bread and white rice), you experience the highs and lows that contribute to storing fat: You get a rush of blood sugar as the carbs are quickly digested, followed by a quick burst of energy, and then a letdown as insulin stores the blood sugar. In turn, your body craves more food—and then eats more.
Attack Plan: Simple. Sub in slow-moving darks for all your fast-acting whites: Choose whole grains and whole wheat products over any made with white flour or refined carbohydrates.

The Heroes: The Flab-Fighting Force

The Hero: Mighty Muscle Man
Given Name: Protein

Primary Superpowers: Helps build muscle and keeps you full and satisfied.
Nutritional Rewards: Protein has more pluses than a math teacher's chalk-board. First of all, protein helps kick-start your metabolism, because your body uses twice as much energy to break down protein as it does to break down car-bohydrates. So when you eat a high-protein meal, you actually burn off addi-tional calories while you're digesting. In one study, people who ate high-protein diets burned more than twice as many calories in the hours after their meals than people who were on high-carbohydrate diets. But protein is also important because it helps flip your satiety switch—you feel fuller faster and longer, mean-ing that you gorge less. Finally, protein serves as the nutritional building block for lean muscle mass. And remember, when you add muscle mass, you're burning even more calories, because your body requires more energy to sustain that mus-cle than it does to sustain fat. Adding 1 pound of muscle equals up to a free 50-calorie burn every day.
Use It: Ideally, you'll integrate protein into all of your meals. You can also eat a little protein—for example, a glass of low-fat milk or a handful of almonds—before your meal. That will help keep your hunger—and portion size—in check.

The Hero: Friendly Fats

Given Name: Polyunsaturated and Monounsaturated Fats

Primary Superpowers: Unclogs arteries and increases satiety.

Nutritional Rewards: We couldn't live without fat any more than we could live without oxygen, water, and Google. We need it to deliver vitamins throughout our bodies, and we need it to produce testosterone—the hormone that leads to muscle growth. We also need it to tag-team with protein to keep us satiated throughout the day. One study showed that dieters who ate modest amounts of fat lost an average of 9 pounds and kept it off a year after the initial 6-month plan, while those on low-fat diets actually regained what they had lost—and then some. Polyunsaturated fats include omega-3 fatty acids that are found in fish like salmon and tuna and help to clear your arteries of bad cholesterol and

---

6-PACK QUIZ

Which fish has the highest amount of omega-3 fatty acids?

    a. Alaska salmon

    b. Pacific herring

    c. Tilapia

    d. Tuna

Answer: b. Pacific herring, which has 2 g per 3-oz serving. The next closest, salmon, has 1.8.

speed your metabolism. Studies show that people who take omega-3s burn more calories throughout the day than those who don't consume those fats. The other kind of good fat—monounsaturated—is found in nuts, olives, avocados, and olive and canola oils. This type also helps reduce bad cholesterol levels and keep you satisfied.

Use It: Sub in olive oil for HFCS-laced salad dressings, or eat a handful of almonds before a meal. And make sure to include a little Friendly Fat at every meal.

The Hero: Carbo-Nator
Given Name: Fiber-Rich Carbohydrates

Primary Superpowers: Slows digestion and the emptying of your stomach so you stay satisfied; provides nutrients for your body.

Nutritional Rewards: Study after study shows that fiber isn't just for backed-up octogenarians. Fiber-rich carbohydrates—remember, the ones with the grains still in them—have all kinds of effects that influence weight loss. Insoluble fiber—your mom used to call it "roughage"—helps pick up fats throughout your digestive system and shuttle them out the door, like a bouncer at spring break. And soluble fiber like that found in oatmeal, apples, and other fruits and grains hangs out in your stomach, where it slows digestion to give you long-burning energy throughout the day. It also helps remove cholesterol from your blood-stream (through a process of binding with digestive acids).

Use It: A high-fiber morning meal has been shown to reduce hunger pangs throughout the day. Get high amounts in oatmeal and whole grain cereal, then use fruits and whole grain breads and pasta as part of your meals.

The Sidekick: Dairy Dude
Given Name: Calcium

Primary Superpowers: Aligns itself with fat-burning properties.
Nutritional Rewards: While calcium is not technically a weight-loss nutrient, more and more research is showing that those who eat calcium experience greater weight loss than those who don't eat it. One Harvard study showed that those people who didn't get the recommended 1,000 milligrams daily were 60 percent more likely to be overweight. And other research shows that calcium can double the rate of weight loss—even when dieters are eating the same number of calories. Researchers aren't sure whether the mineral influences metabolism or

FOODS YOU SHOULD USE

HIGH-QUALITY PROTEIN	SLOW-DIGESTING CARBS	HEALTHY FATS
Eggs and egg whites	Oats	Olive oil
Lean beef	Onions	Canola oil
Turkey	Tomatoes	Fish oil
Chicken	Beans	Flaxseeds
Fish	Green vegetables	Nuts
Fat-free or low-fat milk	Berries	Sunflower seeds
Fat-free or low-fat cheese	Oranges	Olives
Artificially sweetened or sugar-sweetened fat-free or low-fat yogurt	Apples	Avocados

helps restrict daily calories, but there's enough evidence to suggest that calcium may be elevated to hero status very soon.

Use It: The best way to pack in more dairy products without actually touching the udders: a Powerfood smoothie that features low-fat milk or low-fat yogurt. See chapter 7 for recipes.

THE JOY OF ABS

ABS BENEFIT	ABS FACTS
A longer life	Belly fat is the most dangerous kind of fat—it threatens your organs and leads to increases of artery-clogging cholesterol. Losing fat, especially around your belly, improves your health. Studies show that those with the largest waist sizes have increased risk of heart disease and cancer rates. And one study of 8,000 people found that those with the weakest abdominal muscles (an indicator for fattier abdominal regions) had twice the death rate of those with stronger ones.
Less pain	Strong abdominal muscles provide the infrastructure of your body. They play a role in just about every movement you make—whether you're walking, chopping wood, or having sex. Those muscles, along with the ones in your lower back, act as an anatomical girdle or weight belt to give you support throughout the day. Studies show that those people with the strongest abdominal muscles are the least likely to be injured—in all areas of their bodies. And a strong core also helps prevent and alleviate back pain—one of the most common and debilitating injuries for both men and women.

ABS BENEFIT	ABS FACTS
Better sex	Being overweight makes you 50 percent more likely to have sexual dysfunction. One of the major contributors to function: blood supply. When that supply is clogged by fat-related cholesterol, there's less chance for blood to get there. That's true for men and women, since bloodflow influences men's ability to have erections and stimulates women's arousal-sensing and lubricating organs.
More confidence	Seeing your abs is the by-product of an eating and exercise plan that makes you healthy and strong. Those with strong—and visible—abdominal muscles experience increases in self-esteem. Surveys also show that a strong abdominal section is the body part both men and women rate as the most attractive in potential partners.

Chapter 2

THE STRESS/FLAB CONNECTION
Decrease Your Level of Stress
to Decrease the Size of Your Gut

LIKE JUST ABOUT EVERYONE ELSE I know, I'm pretty much stressed out to the max. I have family issues. Work issues. Love life issues. And that Edie on *Desperate Housewives* . . . oh, she makes me so mad!

All this anxiety isn't good for us. You probably already know that stress can raise your blood pressure, diminish your sex drive, and cause excessive horn-blowing in traffic. But did you know it's one of the biggest factors in determining your weight, as well? Here's why.

Stress Changes Your Body

STRESS ISN'T JUST SOMETHING you feel in your head. It's something that trick-les all throughout your body. Under stress, your body produces two hormones: adrenaline and cortisol. Adrenaline is like lighter fluid, and cortisol is like char-coal. The former quickly burns off the immediately available sugar in your blood, so you can fight or flee whatever is stressing you. Cortisol continues to fuel the fire, pumping more sugar into your blood so you have energy to burn. The prob-lem is that excess sugar coursing through your blood is meant to help you flee the saber-toothed tiger or battle the charging wild boar. It's made to be burned off quickly as you either escape or attack. When the stress comes in a more modern form—like a pressing deadline or a stack of unpaid bills—you can't literally fight back or flee. And without that burst of physical activity, you don't have the chance to burn off that extra blood sugar. Instead, it gets stored in your belly as fat.

Every time you feel anxious over those bills or deadlines, there's more mush added around your middle. In a recent study at Yale, women who were most sus-ceptible to stress had both higher levels of cortisol and greater abdominal fat than nonstressed women. And the ladies under stress stored fat primarily in one place: their bellies.

Stress Incites Your Cravings

YOU KNOW THE KID in school who always egged you on to do the things you didn't want to do—throw spitballs, trip the math-club president in the cafeteria, or touch your tongue to the frozen street sign? That's what stress is: the instigator.

It goads you to do things you know aren't good for you, and under pressure, you cave in and do them anyway.

If you reach for chow when you're stressed, it's not because you're weak. It's because you're programmed to do that. Researchers at the University of California, San Francisco, have identified a biochemical feedback system in rats that could explain our stress/craving connection. In their study, the researchers determined that stress stimulated a flood of hormones that prompted the rats to engage in pleasure-seeking behaviors like eating high-calorie foods. While observing pleasure-seeking responses in rats might explain a lot about Charlie Sheen, what does it say about the rest of us? Well, a study done at Yale University found that people with higher stress-induced cortisol levels ate more food—including more sweets—than people with lower cortisol levels.

ABS FACT

41.8

Percent chance that children of overweight parents will turn out the same way

—Journal of Pediatrics

Stress Keeps You—And Your Weight—Up

A UNIVERSITY OF CHICAGO STUDY showed that men who slept only 4 hours a night had cortisol levels 37 percent higher than men who got a full 8 hours. Men who stayed awake the whole night had levels 45 percent higher than the well-rested guys. And remember, increased cortisol equals more fat stored in your belly. Another study tracked the work habits and weights of nearly 1,800 men over a 12-month period and found that those who regularly logged late hours were 36 percent more likely to tip the scales at above-normal weights than the 9-to-5ers.

That's another reason why letting go of stress is an important step toward letting go of pounds. Another University of Chicago study showed that men who were relaxed enough to get deep, quality sleep secreted almost 65 percent more human growth hormone (HGH) than men who didn't fall into deep sleep. Why is HGH important? It helps prevent the loss of muscle mass that can be caused by cortisol. And muscle mass helps you burn calories and maintain a constantly burning metabolism.

Stress Changes Your Decisions

SURE, YOU HAVE EVERY INTENTION of eating right. But when dinner is something that can be considered only in the 15 seconds of free time you have each evening, it's awfully tempting to swing through the drive-thru and pick up something that's ready faster than you can say, "I'll have fries with that." More and more research is showing that a journey to the fast-food emporium is almost as dangerous as a hunting trip with Dick Cheney. Consider:

▶ One study found that fast food increases the risk of obesity and type 2 diabetes. Subjects who consumed fast food just two or more times a week gained about 10 more pounds than participants who consumed fast food less than once per week.

▶ The high-fat, high-carbohydrate content of fast food messes up your blood vessels. A University of Buffalo study found that levels of arterial inflammation remained high for 3 to 4 hours after a high-fat meal. (The study was conducted using an Egg McMuffin and hash browns.)

▶ Soda contains high levels of high-fructose corn syrup, an evil we discussed in chapter 1. On average, we drink 50 gallons of soda per person per year. Yes, you read that right.

▶ Fast and convenient foods are soaked with trans fats. In a 9-year study of more than 16,500 men, researchers found that for every 2 percent increase in trans fat intake, men added one-third of an inch to their waists. (Mono- and polyunsaturated fats had no effect.) Plus, an 80,000-person Harvard study found that getting just 3 percent of your daily calories from trans fats increases your risk of heart disease by up to 50 percent. To put that in perspective, 3 percent of your day's calories totals about 7 grams of trans fats—that's roughly the amount in a single order of fries.

So Now What?

OKAY, SO THIS IS THE POINT in the book where I tell you to relax, not work so hard, and get more sleep. That would also make it the point at which you close

ABS FACT

10 mm/Hg   Amount the average person's diastolic blood pressure increases from ages 30 to 65

—*Journal of the American Medical Association*

the book, hurl it across the room, and start cursing my ancestors. So let's see if we can find a better way, shall we?

Like I said at the top of this chapter, I'm just as stressed as you are. I don't have any magical solutions for finding relaxation and inner peace, and I can't

FIVE FAST STRESS-BUSTERS

Try some of these simple tricks when stress leaves you breathing harder than a bunch of frat brothers at a *Girls Gone Wild* shoot.

▶ **Reward your body.** Regular exercise or relaxation techniques like yoga and massage will keep cortisol naturally in check by releasing beta-endorphins, brain chemicals that give you a calming effect.

▶ **Start strong.** A recent study from Wales shows that regular consumption of breakfast cereal is associated with reduced stress and improved physical and mental health. Those who ate cereal daily had lower levels of cortisol. On the Abs Diet, that means oatmeal and bran cereals.

▶ **Snuff out the midnight oil.** Regularly working overtime may inflate your weight. The stress of a string of 12-hour days can cause a spike in cortisol that stimulates hunger.

▶ **Fight with fish.** That is, integrate more salmon and tuna into your life. When Swiss researchers fortified men's diets with omega-3 fatty acids (fats found in fish), levels of cortisol remained unchanged during stress tests. (The placebo group's cortisol rose by one-third.)

▶ **Get up and get out.** A recent Australian study discovered that workers whose jobs require more than 6 hours of chair time a day are up to 68 percent more likely to wind up overweight or obese.

call your boss, your kids, your spouse, and your creditors and tell them to back off. (Well, I could, but I'd have to charge you a *lot* more for this book.)

Instead, we need to learn to embrace the stress in our lives and start making it work for us. Not to get all new-agey on you (incense is not my thing), but the fact is, we need stress. For example, too much cortisol may force us to gain weight, but too little isn't good for us, either. We need cortisol to help with organ function. Too much stress may make us confused, anxious, and angry, but too little stress makes us bored—and boring.

ABS FACT

68.2

Percentage of US adults who don't get regular leisure-time physical activity

—Weight-Control Information Network

So the point of this book is to help you manage your stress and undo the evils that it can wreak upon you. As long as you have the quick and easy meals and healthy ingredients outlined beginning in chapter 4, you'll have a great weapon with which to battle the ravages of stress. You'll always have healthy food at your fingertips, so you won't be at the mercy of the drive-thru. You'll always be full, so you won't reach for an unhealthy snack when deadlines approach. And you'll have all the food you want in the time you have, so you can get back to what's really important in life—like trying to figure out who's who on *Lost*.

In the following chapters, you'll learn techniques that will help you take control of your time and your food by:

▶ Planning your meals one day at a time, so you can avoid impulsive decisions

▶ Eating six times a day to avoid extreme hunger ups and downs

▶ Making your own meals, so you know exactly what ingredients are being used and, more important, which belly-inflating ones aren't

You *can* fight stress with food. With good food. With Powerfoods. With food that takes less than 6 minutes to make.

THE STRESSED-OUT GUIDE TO QUICK COMFORT FOOD

When you want something chocolatey . . .

Give yourself a fiber edge by picking a candy bar that contains nuts or one that's made with peanut butter. These treats have more of the protein and fiber that will help keep you feeling satisfied.

EAT THIS	NOT THAT
Reese's NutRageous (52 g bar) 280 calories, 6 g protein, 27 g carbs, 16 g total fat, 5 g saturated fat, 105 mg sodium, 2 g fiber	*Kit Kat (42 g bar)* 220 calories, 3 g protein, 27 g carbs, 11 g total fat, 7 g saturated fat, 25 mg sodium, 0 g fiber
OR	OR
Snickers (58.7 g bar) 280 calories, 4 g protein, 35 g carbs, 14 g total fat, 5 g saturated fat, 140 mg sodium, 1 g fiber	*3 Musketeers (60.4 g bar)* 260 calories, 2 g protein, 46 g carbs, 8 g total fat, 5 g saturated fat, 110 mg sodium, 1 g fiber

When you want something piece-y...

Go for something—*anything*—that contains a nutritional component besides sugar; otherwise, you'll just be hungry again in 5 minutes.

EAT THIS	NOT THAT
Peanut M&Ms (1.74 oz) 250 calories, 5 g protein, 30 g carbs, 13 g total fat, 5 g saturated fat, 25 mg sodium, 2 g fiber	*Skittles (2.17 oz)* 250 calories, 0 g protein, 56 g carbs, 2.5 g total fat, 2.5 g saturated fat, 10 mg sodium, 0 g fiber

When you want something crunchy and salty...

There's not a lot to choose from here. Ounce-for-ounce, whole grain Sun Chips offer the most fiber and protein for the least amount of sodium and saturated fat.

EAT THIS	NOT THAT
Sun Chips (1 oz) 140 calories, 2 g protein, 19 g carbs, 6 g total fat, 1 g saturated fat, 115 mg sodium, 2 g fiber	*Cheetos Crunchy (1 oz)* 160 calories, 2 g protein, 15 g carbs, 10 g total fat, 2 g saturated fat, 290 mg sodium, <1 g fiber
OR	OR
Doritos (1 oz) 140 calories, 2 g protein, 17 g carbs, 8 g total fat, 1.5 g saturated fat, 180 mg sodium, 1 g fiber	*Pringles (1 oz)* 160 calories, 1 g protein, 15 g carbs, 11 g total fat, 3 g saturated fat, 170 mg sodium, 1 g fiber

When you want something meaty . . .

Yes, the sodium in beef jerky is off the charts. Oh, well. You're eating in a convenience store. Still, the jerky's lean protein content makes it a smarter snack than one of the hot dogs that's been slowly rotating under a heat lamp for God knows how long.

EAT THIS	NOT THAT
Pemmican Premium Cut Beef Jerky (1 oz) 80 calories, 13 g protein, 4 g carbs, 1 g total fat, 0 g saturated fat, 610 mg sodium, 1 g fiber	*Plain Hot Dog* 280 calories, 11 g protein, 22 g carbs, 17 g total fat, 6 g saturated fat, 710 mg sodium, 1 g fiber

When you want something breakfast-y . . .

Nature Valley's granola bars make a fine breakfast or anytime snack. Four times more protein and double the fiber of most other options. Plus, you get two bars in each packet instead of one.

EAT THIS	NOT THAT
Nature Valley Oats & Honey Bar (2 bars) 180 calories, 4 g protein, 29 g carbs, 6 g total fat, 0.5 g saturated fat, 160 mg sodium, 2 g fiber	*Nutri-Grain Blueberry Bar (1 bar)* 140 calories, 1 g protein, 26 g carbs, 3 g total fat, 0.5 g saturated fat, 105 mg sodium, <1 g fiber

When you want some liquid energy . . .

Despite the claims, there's not much to warrant the promises of most energy drinks . . . except the one claim their packaging obscures: the nearly 30 grams of sugar per can. Go for something that simply boasts caffeine instead; it's a proven energy booster.

DRINK THIS	NOT THAT
Honest T, Black (8 fl oz) 17 calories, 0 g protein, 5 g carbs, 0 g total fat, 0 g saturated fat, 10 mg sodium, 0 g fiber	*Red Bull (8.3 fl oz)* 110 calories, <1 g protein, 28 g carbs, 0 g total fat, 0 g saturated fat, 200 mg sodium, 0 g fiber

When you want something cool and creamy to drink . . .

Quench your thirst *and* your need for gut-busting calcium. The chocolate milk even ekes out a gram of fiber.

DRINK THIS	NOT THAT
Hershey's 1% No Sugar Added Chocolate Milk (8 fl oz) 120 calories, 11 g protein, 15 g carbs, 2.5 g total fat, 2 g saturated fat, 170 mg sodium, 1 g fiber, 60% DV calcium	*Starbucks Frappuccino (9.5 fl oz)* 200 calories, 6 g protein, 37 g carbs, 3 g total fat, 2 g saturated fat, 100 mg sodium, 0 g fiber, 20% DV calcium

When you want something citrusy to drink . . .

Don't be fooled by Sunny D's come-ons. Sure, a 16-ounce bottle contains 200 percent of your daily vitamin C. But the first ingredient is gunky high-fructose corn syrup. Get your C from the source.

DRINK THIS	NOT THAT
Tropicana Pure Premium (14 fl oz) 190 calories, 3 g protein, 43 g carbs, 0 g total fat, 0 g saturated fat, 0 mg sodium, 0 g fiber, 170% DV vitamin C	*Sunny Delight (16 fl oz)* 240 calories, 0 g protein, 58 g carbs, 0 g total fat, 0 g saturated, 380 mg sodium, 0 g fiber, 200% DV vitamin C

VITAMINS, SEE?

VITAMINS are nature's medicine. Eating foods that contain an alphabet's worth of vitamins is like getting a lifetime subscription to a healthier body. Turn the page for details about the vitamins your body craves.

VITAMIN	BASIC JOBS	THE LATEST
Vitamin A	Protects eyesight Boosts immunity Protects and maintains skin	The latest research has focused on vitamin A's ability to treat acne—but this hasn't involved the nutrient's dietary form. (You probably don't want to suck down a tube of OxyClear anyway.) Vitamin A is a carotenoid, and there have been recent developments on its precursor form, beta-carotene. (See page 50 for more on that.)
Vitamin B_6	Boosts immunity Manufactures protein for body cells Carries oxygen to cells via bloodstream Regulates blood sugar Reduces risk of heart disease	High levels of vitamin B_6 may reduce the risk of colon cancer in women, according to a recent Harvard Medical School study. When researchers tested blood levels of B_6 against rates of cancer, they found that those women with high levels of the vitamin were 44 percent less likely to develop colorectal cancer and 58 percent less likely to develop colon cancer. B_6 appears to prevent cancer-causing damage to DNA.

AMOUNT YOU NEED DAILY	WHERE TO GET IT
900 International Units (IU) for men 700 IU for women	1 cup cooked pumpkin: 54,037 IU 1 cup cooked carrots: 38,304 IU 1 baked sweet potato (with skin): 31,860 IU 1 cup raw carrots: 30,942 IU 1 baked sweet potato (without skin): 26,604 IU 1 cup canned mixed vegetables: 18,985 IU 1 cup cooked spinach: 14,742 IU 1 cup cooked turnip greens: 13,079 IU 1 cup cooked collard greens: 10,168 IU 1 cup cooked kale: 9,620 IU 1 cup red bell pepper: 8,493 IU 1 mango: 8,061 IU 1 cup cooked butternut squash: 8,014 IU 1 cup canned chicken vegetable soup: 5,878 IU 1 cup diced cantaloupe: 5,411 IU
1.3 mg	1 serving heavily fortified cereal (such as Total): 2 mg ½ cup All Bran: 1.8 mg 3 oz cooked yellowfin tuna: 0.89 mg 1 packet fortified instant oats: 0.74 mg 1 cup enriched rice: 0.64 mg 1 baked potato (with skin): 0.62 mg 1 cup dried plums: 0.54 mg 3 oz chicken breast meat: 0.52 mg 1 serving lightly fortified cereal (such as Cheerios): 0.50 mg 1 oz pistachios: 0.48 mg 1 baked potato (without skin): 0.47 mg 3 oz turkey breast meat: 0.45 mg 1 banana: 0.40 mg

(continued)

VITAMIN	BASIC JOBS	THE LATEST
Vitamin B$_{12}$	Builds red blood cells Forms DNA Reduces risk of heart disease	Calcium gets all the press for preventing osteoporosis, but vitamin B$_{12}$ may also help your bones stay snap-free. When scientists with the USDA's Agricultural Research Service recently compared levels of the vitamin to markers of bone health in 2,576 men and women, they found that people with the highest levels of B$_{12}$ also had the highest bone density. A study from Tufts University found that high levels of B$_{12}$ improved bone density by 7 percent, on average. Vitamin B$_{12}$ helps build new bone cells.
Vitamin C (aka ascorbic acid)	Boosts immunity Protects all cells from free-radical damage Heals wounds Prevents bruising Lowers blood pressure	After years of flip-flopping research, a recent study suggests that taking vitamin C supplements regularly can cut your chances of coming down with a cold. When scientists from Japan's National Cancer Center supplied 244 men and women with either 50 mg vitamin C or 500 mg vitamin C, to be taken daily for 5 years, the people in the high-C group experienced an average of four fewer colds than the low-C group.

AMOUNT YOU NEED DAILY	WHERE TO GET IT
2.4 mcg	6 raw oysters: 16 mcg 1 cup canned clam chowder: 10 mcg 3 oz cooked king crab: 10 mcg 1 serving heavily fortified cereal (such as Total): 6 mcg 3 oz cooked sockeye salmon: 5 mcg 3 oz cooked rainbow trout: 4 mcg 3 oz canned salmon: 4 mcg 3 oz smoked salmon: 3 mcg 3 oz steamed/boiled lobster meat: 3 mcg 3 oz canned tuna: 3 mcg 1 typical fast-food cheeseburger: 3 mcg 3 oz cooked beef tenderloin: 2 mcg 1 cup typical tuna salad: 2 mcg 3 oz cooked ground beef (75–80% lean): 2 mcg 3 oz cooked lamb: 2 mcg
90 mg for men/75 mg for women; however, many experts recommend higher levels (250–500 mg)	1 cup red bell pepper: 283 mg 1 papaya: 188 mg 1 cup green bell pepper: 133 mg 1 cup orange juice (fresh-squeezed): 124 mg 1 cup cooked broccoli: 116 mg 1 hot red or green chile pepper: 109 mg 1 cup orange juice (from frozen): 97 mg 1 cup strawberries: 97 mg 1 cup cooked Brussels sprouts: 96 mg 1 cup grapefruit juice (white or pink): 94 mg 8 oz cranberry juice cocktail: 90 mg 1 cup raw broccoli: 82 mg 1 cup cooked peas: 76 mg 1 kiwifruit: 70 mg 1 orange: 70 mg

(continued)

VITAMIN	BASIC JOBS	THE LATEST
Vitamin D	Boosts calcium absorption Builds and maintains bones and teeth Boosts immunity Fights colon cancer	Vitamin D may score an "A" when it comes to helping men prevent prostate cancer. In a recent lab study, researchers from the University of Rochester Medical Center found that the sunshine vitamin can inhibit the spread of prostate cancer cells by limiting the activity of two specific enzymes, proteases called matrix metalloproteinase and cathepsin. Shutting down these enzymes limits cancer cells' ability to invade healthy cells.
Vitamin E	Protects all cells from free-radical damage Controls blood sugar	Science has come down hard on vitamin E recently, determining that its claims for cancer and heart disease prevention are overblown. While those diseases may be top killers, they're not the only ones that could cause you to check out early. Researchers from Harvard recently found that vitamin E may help protect against amyotrophic lateral sclerosis, aka Lou Gehrig's disease. They found that people with high levels of vitamin E were 62 percent less likely to develop the degenerative neurological disorder.

AMOUNT YOU NEED DAILY	WHERE TO GET IT
200 IU for ages 31–50 400 IU for ages 51–70	3 oz canned salmon: 530 IU 3.5 oz cooked salmon: 360 IU 3.5 oz cooked mackerel: 345 IU 3 oz tuna canned in oil: 200 IU 1 cup fortified fat-free milk: 100 IU 1 cup fortified orange juice: 100 IU ½ cup pudding (fortified or prepared with fortified milk): 50 IU 1 serving heavily fortified cereal (such as Total): 40 IU 1 egg: 20 IU 1 oz Swiss cheese: 12 IU Vitamin D is hard to come by in foods. Fifteen minutes of sunlight also will supply the amount you need each day.
15 mg	1 serving heavily fortified cereal (such as Total): 14 mg ¼ cup sunflower seeds: 12 mg 1 oz almonds: 6 mg 1 Tbsp sunflower oil: 5 mg 1 Tbsp safflower oil: 5 mg 1 cup tomato sauce: 5 mg 1 cup cooked spinach: 5 mg 1 cup cooked turnip greens: 4 mg 1 oz mixed nuts: 3 mg 1 cup soymilk: 3 mg 1 cup canned pumpkin: 3 mg 1 cup cooked or canned sweet potato (without skin): 3 mg 1 cup cooked broccoli: 3 mg 1 cup red bell pepper: 2 mg 1 Tbsp canola, corn, or soybean oil: 2 mg

(continued)

VITAMIN	BASIC JOBS	THE LATEST
Beta-carotene	Protects eyesight Boosts immunity	Beta-carotene is like an edible sunscreen. National Cancer Institute researchers have found that people with the highest intakes of carotenoids like beta-carotene are six times less likely to develop skin cancer than those with low intakes. The vitamin plants itself in your skin cells, where its imperceptible orange and yellow pigments help deflect harmful sunlight.
Folate (aka folic acid)	Fights cancer Prevents heart disease Builds new cells throughout the body	Researchers at the University of California, Irvine, found that people who consumed 400 mcg folate daily decreased their risk of developing Alzheimer's disease by 55 percent. Researchers speculate that folate helps you stay sharp for life by controlling homocysteine, an amino acid that can damage nerve cells.

AMOUNT YOU NEED DAILY	WHERE TO GET IT
3,000–6,000 mcg	1 cup canned pumpkin: 17,003 mcg
	1 baked sweet potato (with skin): 16,803 mcg
	1 cup cooked spinach: 13,750 mcg
	1 cup cooked carrots: 12,998 mcg
	1 cup cooked collard greens: 11,591 mcg
	1 cup cooked kale: 11,470 mcg
	1 cup cooked turnip greens: 10,593 mcg
	1 cup canned mixed vegetables: 9,242 mcg
	1 cup raw carrots: 9,114 mcg
	1 cup cooked winter squash: 5,726 mcg
	1 cup cooked Chinese cabbage (bok choy): 4,333 mcg
	1 cup cantaloupe: 3,232 mcg
	1 cup cooked red bell pepper: 3,040 mcg
	1 cup canned vegetable soup: 2,875 mcg
	1 cup raw red bell pepper: 2,420 mcg
400 mcg	1 cup enriched rice: 767 mcg
	1 serving heavily fortified cereal (such as Total): 676 mcg
	1 serving All Bran: 659 mcg
	1 cup cooked lentils: 358 mcg
	1 cup cooked black-eyed peas: 358 mcg
	1 serving lightly fortified cereal (such as Wheaties): 336 mcg
	1 cup cooked pinto beans: 294 mcg
	1 cup cooked chickpeas: 282 mcg
	1 cup cooked okra: 269 mcg
	1 cup cooked spinach: 263 mcg
	1 cup cooked black beans: 256 mcg
	1 cup cooked asparagus: 243 mcg
	1 cup cooked kidney beans: 230 mcg
	1 cup fortified oatmeal: 199 mcg
	1 cup cooked collard greens: 177 mcg

CRANK UP THE HEAVY METAL!

VITAMINS GET ALL THE PRESS, but minerals are just as important for keeping your body functioning at its highest level. Turn the page for details about the precious metals you need more of.

MINERAL	BASIC JOBS	THE LATEST
Calcium	Builds and maintains bones and teeth Regulates muscle contraction Transmits nerve impulses	Recent research from the University of Tennessee found that eating yogurt can help you lose weight—specifically, by zapping the flab from your gut. In the 12-week study, people who consumed about three 6-ounce servings of fat-free yogurt daily lost 81 percent more fat from their midsections than those who ate a variety of dairy products containing less total calcium. The belly-busting effect may come from calcium's effect on the stress hormone cortisol, according to researchers. The mineral appears to help curb production of this hormone that has been linked to the accumulation of abdominal fat.
Iron	Carries oxygen to cells via bloodstream Energizes muscles	Most nutrition-disease links involve deficiencies—you don't obtain enough of a certain mineral or vitamin, and you develop a related disease. With iron, the opposite is true, as illustrated by recent research from the University of Washington, Seattle. When scientists compared diets of people recently diagnosed with Parkinson's disease to those of people without it, they found that people with the highest levels of iron in their diets were 1.7 times more likely to be Parkinson's patients than those with the lowest intakes. Too much iron can cause oxidative stress, a situation where cells release toxic substances called free radicals. That oxidation may cause degeneration of brain cells that produce dopamine—the same cells that are affected by Parkinson's, say researchers. Iron overload is especially dangerous for men; because premenopausal women menstruate, their iron levels are kept in check.

AMOUNT YOU NEED DAILY	**WHERE TO GET IT**
1,000 mg	1 serving heavily fortified cereal (such as Total): 1,000 mg 8 oz low-fat yogurt: 415 mg 4 oz tofu: 434 mg 1 cup cooked collard greens: 266 mg ½ cup reduced-fat ricotta cheese: 337 mg 1 cup fat-free milk: 301 mg 1 cup fortified orange juice: 300 mg 1 oz low-fat Swiss cheese: 272 mg 1 cup edamame: 261 mg 1 cup cooked turnip greens: 249 mg 1 oz provolone cheese: 214 mg 1 cup cooked black-eyed peas: 211 mg 1 oz reduced-fat mozzarella cheese: 207 mg 1 typical fast-food cheeseburger: 206 mg 1 oz Cheddar cheese: 204 mg
8 mg for men 18 mg for women	3 oz clams: 24 mg 1 serving heavily fortified cereal (such as raisin bran, corn flakes, or Total): 18 mg 1 cup baked beans (with pork): 8 mg 1 cup enriched white rice: 8 mg 1 serving lightly fortified cereal (such as Cheerios, Chex, Crispix): 8 mg 1 cup canned white beans: 8 mg 1 cup canned kidney beans: 6 mg 1 cup lentils: 6 mg 1 cup cooked spinach: 6 mg 1 packet enriched instant oatmeal: 6 mg 1 typical fast-food hamburger: 5 mg 1 cup chickpeas: 4 mg 3 oz beef tenderloin: 3 mg ½ cup trail mix (with chocolate chips): 3 mg 3 oz tuna canned in water: 3 mg

(continued)

MINERAL	BASIC JOBS	THE LATEST
Magnesium	Builds and maintains bones and teeth Relaxes muscles after contraction Initiates heartbeat Regulates blood pressure	Eating foods high in magnesium could keep your colon clear of cancer. In a recent study, researchers from the University of Minnesota found that people whose diets include at least 356 mg magnesium daily were 25 percent less likely to develop colon cancer. Aside from the fact that foods containing magnesium tend to be high in fiber (another nutrient linked to colon cancer prevention), researchers suggest that magnesium may also help reduce oxidative stress and cancer cell proliferation.
Potassium	Maintains proper fluid balance Regulates muscle contraction Transmits nerve impulses Helps lower blood pressure	In a Harvard School of Public Health study of almost 44,000 men, researchers found that those whose diets were rich in potassium had a 38 percent lower risk of stroke than those whose diets contained less of the mineral. Although potassium has been shown to help lower blood pressure (high BP is a cause of stroke), the Harvard researchers believe that the stroke-prevention benefit is independent of BP regulation. That means potassium may have other as-yet-undiscovered abilities to stop stroke.

AMOUNT YOU NEED DAILY	WHERE TO GET IT
400 mg for men ages 19–30 420 mg for men ages 31+ 310 mg for women ages 19–30 320 mg for women ages 31+	½ cup wheat germ: 275 mg 1 cup cooked spinach: 156 mg 1 oz roasted pumpkin seeds: 151 mg ¼ cup sunflower seeds: 127 mg 1 cup cooked black beans: 120 mg ½ cup trail mix (with chocolate chips): 118 mg 4 oz tofu: 118 mg 1 cup cooked white beans: 113 mg ½ skinless turkey breast: 109 mg 1 cup cooked artichokes: 101 mg 1 cup cooked lima beans: 101 mg 1 cup cooked okra: 94 mg 3 oz halibut: 90 mg 1 oz almonds: 86 mg 1 cup cooked pinto beans: 70 mg
4,700 mg daily	½ skinless turkey breast: 1,142 mg 1 cup cooked white beans: 1,004 mg 1 cup edamame: 970 mg 1 cup cooked lima beans: 955 mg 1 cup tomato sauce: 909 mg 1 cup cooked winter squash: 896 mg 1 baked potato: 844 mg 1 cup cooked spinach: 839 mg 1 papaya: 781 mg ½ avocado: 742 mg 1 cup cooked lentils: 731 mg 1 cup cooked kidney beans: 717 mg ½ cup raisins: 543 mg 8 oz low-fat yogurt: 497 mg 1 cup cooked pinto beans: 495 mg

(continued)

MINERAL	BASIC JOBS	THE LATEST
Selenium	Protects all cells from free-radical damage Boosts immunity Protects prostate gland Regulates thyroid gland function	University of North Carolina at Chapel Hill researchers recently found that having higher selenium levels may reduce your risk of developing osteoarthritis. When researchers compared blood levels of the mineral to knee x-rays that illustrated cartilage erosion in nearly 1,000 people, they discovered that those people with higher selenium concentrations were nearly half as likely to develop arthritis in their knee joints. In your body, selenium has an antioxidant effect, helping to tamp down the inflammation associated with arthritis.
Zinc	Manufactures testosterone Boosts immunity Heals wounds Maintains sense of taste and smell Protects eyesight	Eating more of this mineral may help you move more metal. In a small study, researchers from the USDA's Agricultural Research Service compared exercise performance in men with low and high zinc concentrations. After exercise, the guys whose diets contained more zinc showed improved peak oxygen uptake, carbon dioxide output, and respiratory exchange ratio. Zinc helps red blood cells remove carbon dioxide from the blood—making more room for oxygen.

AMOUNT YOU NEED DAILY	WHERE TO GET IT
55 mcg	1 oz Brazil nuts: 544 mcg
	1 oz mixed nuts: 119 mcg
	1 cup typical tuna salad: 85 mcg
	3 oz tuna canned in water: 68 mcg
	6 raw oysters: 54 mcg
	3 oz swordfish: 53 mcg
	3 oz flounder: 50 mcg
	3 oz perch: 47 mcg
	1 cup typical chili: 44 mcg
	1 cup cooked enriched rice: 43 mcg
	1 cup couscous: 43 mcg
	3 oz ham: 42 mcg
	3.5 oz cooked beef: 35 mcg
	3 oz turkey breast meat: 27 mcg
	3 oz chicken breast meat: 23 mcg
11 mg for men	6 raw oysters: 76 mg
8 mg for women	1 serving heavily fortified cereal (such as Total): 15 mg
	1 cup baked beans (with pork): 15 mg
	3 oz cooked beef, chuck roast: 9 mg
	1 serving lightly fortified cereal (such as Wheaties): 7 mg
	3 oz cooked king crab: 6 mg
	3 oz cooked lamb: 6 mg
	3 oz cooked beef, sirloin: 5 mg
	1 cup typical chili: 5 mg
	1 typical fast-food roast beef sandwich: 4 mg
	3 oz cooked beef, ground (80–95% lean): 4 mg
	1 cup baked beans: 4 mg
	1 cup reduced-fat ricotta: 3 mg

Chapter 3

THE ABS DIET ARSENAL

The Six Easy Guidelines That Will Make You Lean for Life

IF YOU ASK ME, RULES CAN BE QUITE USEFUL for toddlers, felons, and whiz-where-they-want pets. When it comes to dieting, however, I think rules have about the same long-term effect on weight loss as banana splits—they just don't work.

Too many diets are about deprivation. And let's face it: Once you're told you can't have something, man oh man, don't you just want it more? So in the Abs Diet, I want you to stop thinking you have rules. I want you to simply rethink the way you eat. Follow the guidelines in this chapter, and you'll feel what it's like to eat right, stay satisfied, and fuel your body with high-octane energy. In just a few days, you'll have changed the rules of weight loss so that there are none—there's only your new approach to eating, the one that will help burn your fat, build your muscle, and give you options to stay lean for life.

Because I believe abs, beer, and Star Wars movies aren't the only good things that come in sixes, I've developed six guidelines that provide the foundation for the Abs Diet eating system. Follow the Abs Diet ways of eating, and you'll be able to ditch the old rules—as well as your old body.

The Old Diet Way: Eat breakfast, lunch, and dinner.

The Abs Diet Way: Eat six times a day.

OLD DIET SYSTEMS want you to stay hungry by forcing you to eat a daily calorie count that's lower than Jessica Simpson's SAT scores. I don't want you hungry—I want you full. When you're full, you won't be as tempted (or likely) to steamroll your way through pizza boxes, chips bags, and your neighbor's pantry. And the way you'll get full: Eat six times a day with a variety of the nutritional heroes outlined in chapter 1. By eating every few hours, you keep your metabolism revved and ensure overall stomach satisfaction. Now, there's a big difference between "satisfaction" and "gluttony." But the great thing about the Abs Diet Powerfoods is that they come with their own appetite-regulation system. Because the Powerfoods are high in nutrients, protein, healthy fats, and fiber, it's almost impossible to overeat. Proper nutrition will leave you feeling satiated all day long.

HOW TO DO IT: Eat three standard meals with three smaller snacks. For example:

> 8 a.m.: Breakfast
>
> 11 a.m.: Snack
>
> 1 p.m.: Lunch
>
> 4 p.m.: Snack
>
> 6 p.m.: Dinner
>
> 9 p.m.: Snack

The Old Diet Way: Deprive yourself of specific foods.

The Abs Diet Way: Indulge in specific foods—the Abs Diet Power 12.

MOST DIETS TREAT YOU as if you're the kid and they're the parent: no this, no that, no fruit, no bread, no meat, no potatoes, no sugar, no, no, no, no. And you end up hearing no more often than the science club president 3 weeks before the prom. Yes, it's true that there are foods and substances so toxic that you should stiff-arm them like Tiki Barber shaking off a tackler. But there's an enormous world of wonderful foods out there just waiting for you. And it's not all veggies and tofu; the preferred foods are as diverse in their taste as they are in their nutritional power. Adopt the Abs Diet Power 12. Eat the Abs Diet Power 12. Enjoy the Abs Diet Power 12.

HOW TO DO IT: Make sure that every meal includes at least two foods from the Powerfoods list, but try to make meals in which every food is a Powerfood. The more you use the foods, the better your results.

The Old Diet Way: No dessert for you!

The Abs Diet Way: Have dessert EVERY day!

IN FACT, I INSIST. If you want to really start dropping pounds, a sweet, creamy Abs Diet smoothie for dessert—any night or every night if you want—is a great step in the right direction.

Let's face it: There's a basic human need for sweets. It comes from our days as scavengers, when our taste buds encouraged us to seek out berries and other fruits, helping ensure that we got all the vitamins and minerals we needed. Today, we still crave sweets: We crave them when we're stressed. We reach for them when we're tired. We feel for them at the end of the meal. And to completely eliminate sweets from your life goes against human nature and guarantees only one thing—dietary failure.

So how can you fulfill your sweet cravings but not blow a week's worth of calories on a chain-restaurant cake that's the size of an ottoman? With a powerful and sweet Abs Diet smoothie. In each drink, you can get the taste of chocolate, or berries, or pumpkin—without the guilt that typically comes from desserts. Packed with Powerfoods, smoothies will also take up valuable stomach space, so you avoid the blood sugar highs and lows associated with desserts filled with simple sugars.

(continued on page 70)

ABS DIET POWER 12

Abs

POWERFOOD	IMPORTANCE	EAT 'EM	FORGET 'EM	HOW TO USE 'EM
A: Almonds and other nuts	Nuts and seeds contain protein and monounsaturated fats that help you feel full. And almonds contain magnesium that helps you build muscle.	Almonds, peanuts, Brazil nuts, cashews, hazelnuts, pecans, pine nuts, pumpkin seeds, sunflower seeds	Smoked and salted nuts, candy-coated nuts	Eat about 24 almonds a day—that's about two handfuls. That amount won't lead to weight gain and should suppress your appetite, making it a good late-afternoon snack.
B: Beans and legumes	They're packed with protein, iron, and fiber, which help you build muscle and lose weight.	Soybeans, pinto beans, chickpeas, navy beans, black beans, white beans, kidney beans, lima beans, green beans, lentils, peas, hummus, edamame	Refried beans, which are high in saturated fat, and baked beans, which are high in sugar	Sub black beans for ground beef in meat-heavy dishes to eliminate saturated fats and add fiber.
S: Spinach and other green vegetables	Green vegetables, especially spinach, have the vitamin power to protect you against heart attack and stroke. Broccoli is loaded with calcium and vitamin C.	Spinach, broccoli, Brussels sprouts, asparagus, peppers, some lettuces, avocados	Iceberg lettuce (contains few vitamins and little fiber, unlike romaine or arugula)	If you don't like veggies, mask them in chili, or add a few to a chicken stir-fry with olive oil and garlic.

(continued)

ABS DIET POWER 12 (CONT.)

Diet

POWERFOOD	IMPORTANCE	EAT 'EM	FORGET 'EM	HOW TO USE 'EM
D: Dairy (fat-free or low-fat milk, yogurt, cheese)	Calcium has been shown to be a key ingredient in weight loss. Used as a base for smoothies, low-fat milk provides volume to keep your stomach full and satisfied.	Milk, yogurt, cheese, cottage cheese	Whole milk (high in fat), frozen yogurt (high in sugar)	Drink a glass of 2% milk before dinner to help take up some room in your stomach.
I: Instant oatmeal (unsweetened, unflavored)	Oatmeal contains soluble fiber that helps lower your cholesterol. In one study, it was shown to sustain blood-sugar levels longer than any other food, making sure you won't be ravenous in a few hours.	Other high-fiber cereals	Oatmeal with sugar or high-fructose corn syrup	Add a little cooked oatmeal to a smoothie for increased fiber. Nuke oatmeal with frozen berries and 1% milk for a good after-dinner snack.

POWERFOOD	IMPORTANCE	EAT 'EM	FORGET 'EM	HOW TO USE 'EM
E: Eggs	The protein found in eggs is more effective for building muscle than is protein from other sources. (Eating an egg or two won't raise cholesterol levels.)	Eggs, egg whites	The "everything" omelet at the diner	For a fast breakfast, mix two eggs in a bowl and microwave on high for 60 to 90 seconds, until set. You'll have instant scrambled eggs.
T: Turkey and other lean meats	Eating protein means your body will burn more calories (it uses more calories to burn protein than to burn fats or carbs). Plus, it helps build fat-burning muscle. Split your meats so that you usually have lean meats like fish and poultry, with occasional portions of red meat. Fish has polyunsaturated fats, and chicken and turkey have lean protein to build muscle.	Turkey, chicken, fish (especially salmon and tuna), shellfish, Canadian bacon, lean steak like extra-lean ground beef, tenderloin, London broil, flank steak	Sausage, bacon, cured meats, ham, fatty cuts of steak	Don't like fish? Eat flaxseed—ground or oil. One teaspoon of ground flaxseed has only 60 calories, but it contains 4 grams of fiber and is loaded with omega-3s. Sprinkle into oatmeal or smoothies.

(continued)

ABS DIET POWER 12 *(CONT.)*

Power! POWERFOOD	IMPORTANCE	EAT 'EM	FORGET 'EM	HOW TO USE 'EM
P: Peanut butter	It contains monounsaturated fats that have been shown to help keep you full. It's also a sinful-tasting food that can add variety and taste to a diet.	PB that's all-natural and sugar-free, almond butter	Sugary brands or trans fatty peanut butters	Limit yourself to 3 tablespoons a day because of high fat content. Perfect snack: PB on whole wheat toast with crushed berries
O: Olive oil	With the same monounsaturated fats as peanut butter, it'll help control your cravings.	Olive oil, canola oil, peanut oil, sesame oil	Vegetable and hydrogenated vegetable oils, trans fatty acids, margarine	Drip a little on vegetables, salad, even rice or a baked potato
W: Whole grain breads and cereals	The unrefined parts that contain nutrients and fiber remain. All-white breads and pasta don't include those fiber-rich elements to help your digestive system. Whole grain foods keep insulin levels low, so you're less likely to store fat.	Whole grain bread, whole grain cereal, brown rice, whole wheat pretzels, whole wheat pasta	White bread, bagels, doughnuts, breads labeled as "wheat" instead of "whole wheat"	Buy whole wheat pasta with flaxseed for a double punch of power.

POWERFOOD	IMPORTANCE	EAT 'EM	FORGET 'EM	HOW TO USE 'EM
E: Extra-protein (whey) powder	Whey protein is a high-quality protein containing amino acids that build muscle and burn fat. It has the highest amount of protein for the fewest calories.	Whey powder, ricotta cheese	Soy protein	Drink a smoothie before a workout. One study showed it helped increase strength better than drinking one after a workout.
R: Raspberries and other berries	Berries have cancer-fighting antioxidants and contain fiber to help you feel fuller longer.	Raspberries, blueberries, strawberries, cranberries, and other fruits like apples	Jelly	Blueberries are tops in antioxidants and loaded with soluble fiber.

ABS FACT

Research shows that having high weight-loss goals will help you lose a greater amount of weight. Researchers found that those people who tried to lose an average of 16 percent of their body weight—instead of the commonly recommended 5 to 10 percent—dropped more weight than those who were more conservative.

HOW TO DO IT: Follow the recipes in this book, in *The Abs Diet,* or in *The Abs Diet Eat Right Every Time Guide.* Use smoothies as snacks or as replacement meals.

> **The Old Diet Way: Count every calorie, or weigh every portion, or assign points to each food, or eat your meals in some sort of "zone."**
>
> **The Abs Diet Way: Have a life.**

SURE, SOME OF US are obsessive-compulsive math geeks or NASA rocket scientists. We need to account for every calorie we consume and every calorie we burn so we can calculate our optimum payload and energy expenditure. That's fine if it works for you. But you know what? Most of us have our hands so full with work, kids, and *CSI* reruns that we don't have the time to make eating right more complicated than air-traffic control. I believe that the only way most of us will stick to an eating plan long-term is if we strip away the difficulties of it. So, on the Abs Diet, there will be no counting calories or fat grams. Eat the Power 12, and the calories will take care of themselves.

HOW TO DO IT: Eat meals balanced with different nutrients—making sure to include stomach-satisfying high-fiber whole grains, good fats, and protein. Let your foods do the counting.

> ## The Old Diet Way: It's the food, stupid.
>
> ## The Abs Diet Way: It's the drink, stupid.

YOUR FOOD INTAKE can be as healthy and as disciplined as a monk, and you can still be consuming too many calories. Between high-sugar OJ, high-fat whole milk, high-calorie sports drinks, and higher-calorie Budweisers, it's scary how many unhealthy fats and carbohydrates you can consume without ever biting into anything. For that reason, I want you to really examine what you drink along with and between your meals.

FREQUENTLY ABS QUESTIONS

WHAT SHOULD I EAT TO TREAT A HANGOVER?

Oatmeal. When researchers from Wales gave breakfasts to hungover college students (now there's a job I'd pass on), those students who ate a meal of slowly digestible carbohydrates fared better on mood and memory tests than those who had simple sugars (think Fruity Pebbles).

HOW TO DO IT: Drink water, fat-free or low-fat milk, and smoothies. Coffee and tea are okay, too. But avoid whole-fat dairy products and high-sugar fruit juices. Alcohol? Best to limit yourself to two or three drinks per week, because you don't need the extra calories, although many studies have shown that alcohol has many benefits when consumed in moderation (one to two drinks a day). Though the verdict is out on diet drinks, I'd recommend avoiding them because some research shows that they may contribute to weight gain (by triggering you to feel hungry). And for goodness sake, stop with the soda. For all our talk about less exercise and more fast food, our constantly increasing soda consumption (50 gallons per person per year!) may well be the biggest reason of all why America is facing an obesity epidemic.

FREQUENTLY ABS QUESTIONS

IS IT OKAY TO DRINK DIET SODA?

Even though it has fewer calories than celery, diet soda may not turn out to be the weight-loss savior everyone thinks it is. In fact, drinking diet soda may actually raise your risk of becoming fat. A University of Texas study showed that people who drank at least one diet soda a day had a 55-percent chance of being overweight—a 22-percent difference over regular cola drinkers. Researchers theorize that the diet soda's sweet taste might prime your body to expect a large number of calories, causing you to crave—and consume—other, high-calorie foods.

TURN BAD FOODS GOOD

How to Make Some of Life's Nastiest Ingredients Nutritious

BAD FOODS	TURNED GOOD
Burger. Some ground beef is loaded with lots of fat, and the white-bread bun has next to no nutritional value.	Use extra-lean beef, and mix in chopped onions and chopped frozen spinach. You can even use lean ground buffalo to reduce the fat intake.
Sausage-and-egg biscuit. Sausage patties and biscuits drip with saturated and trans fats.	Nuke a beaten egg on high for 60 to 90 seconds, until set, then use much leaner Canadian bacon. Serve it over a whole wheat English muffin.
Grilled cheese. You'll get 18 grams of saturated fat from the butter and slabs of oily cheese.	Whole wheat bread with reduced-fat mozzarella in between. Crisp it in a pan using a little olive oil.
Nachos. About 12 chips contain 120 calories—and that's not even including the cheese, sour cream, and greasy meat.	Use baked corn chips, pinto beans, extra-lean ground beef, and reduced-fat sharp Cheddar. Top it with some tomatoes and onions.

The Old Diet Way: Don't cheat.

The Abs Diet Way: Cheat like Jude Law at a nanny convention.

DIETS USED TO BE like marriages: If you strayed from the rules, you were done. You cheated. Forget it. Diet's over.

But I want you to cheat (on the diet, that is). One meal a week, I want you to eat whatever you want. Beer and chicken wings? Sure. Double-stuffed pizza and a Big Gulp? Indulge. Battered swine intestines and goat's milk? Hey, whatever dunks your doughnut. Whatever you choose, you're doing it for a reason: because you never want to feel deprived. Deprivation leads to resentment, which leads to your having an ongoing secret affair with both Ben *and* Jerry. But if you pick one meal a week in which there are no holds barred, you'll feel in control for the rest of the week—like eating healthy is your choice, not your chore.

HOW TO DO IT: Pick one weekly meal when you want to blow it out—and then blow it out. My suggestion: Time it to a party, a poker game, or your office happy hour. (Many Abs Diet devotees say that they don't even feel like doing the cheat meal after the first week or two, because their bodies have adjusted so well to the Powerfoods that they don't feel the need to cheat.)

HOW TO READ A NUTRITION LABEL

THE WORDING	THE INSIDE STORY	BOTHER LOOKING?
Serving Size and Servings Per Container	What you think is one serving actually may be two—especially with bottled beverages, like iced tea, colas, and sports drinks. The "100" calories on the label could actually mean 200 for the whole bottle.	Yes. Read first to see how much that bottle, pack, or box is worth.
Calories	Calories can be an arbitrary reading, because everyone's caloric needs are different.	Don't count calories, but it's always smart to be aware of foods that are extremely caloric. If you stick to the Powerfoods, you won't have to obsess over calories, because the foods will keep you full.
Calories from Fat	If you multiply this number by 3 and get a number nearly as big as total calories, it means the food is laced with fat. Next step: Scan for total fat.	Yes, for that quick calculation.

(continued)

THE WORDING	THE INSIDE STORY	BOTHER LOOKING?
Total Fat	Total of all fats—the good (monounsaturated and polyunsaturated) and the bad (saturated and trans).	Look, but don't be misled. Unless you're talking about pageant contestants, a high fat content isn't always a bad thing. You want a higher proportion of the good fats than the bad ones.
% Daily Value	It's the percentage of daily intake the food supplies, based on a 2,000-calorie-a-day diet.	You're not counting calories. Ignore it.
Cholesterol	It represents the amount of cholesterol in the food, but it's not that important, since your body, not your food, manufactures most of your cholesterol.	Don't sweat it. If you want to ballpark it, shoot for 300 mg or less a day.
Sodium	It's a mineral added for flavor and to help preserve foods. They're typically big numbers, but don't panic.	Unless you have high blood pressure or are salt-sensitive, use 2,000 mg per day as a reasonable target.
Total Carbohydrates	All of the sugar, starch, and fiber in a food. The total isn't what's important. The ratio is.	Nope. Look farther down to the ratio of carbs (fiber versus sugars).

THE WORDING	THE INSIDE STORY	BOTHER LOOKING?
Dietary Fiber	It's the roughage that keeps your digestive system flowing—in the form of both soluble fiber (which keeps blood vessels lubed) and insoluble fiber (which is digested but not absorbed, to keep you feeling fuller longer).	Any food with more than 2 g is good.
Sugars	Any and all kinds—from fruit sugars, to dairy sugars, to refined sugars. And it also includes the killers—sucrose (table sugar) and high-fructose corn syrup.	Aim for 5 g or less of sugar per serving.
Protein	The amino acids that build and maintain your body.	You don't need to keep track of it. Most Americans get plenty of protein a day.
Vitamin and Mineral Percentages	All labels include four (vitamins A and C, calcium, and iron).	Ignore it. Take a multivitamin every day to take care of your overall vitamin needs rather than trying to piece together totals with every food.

Chapter 4

6-PACK BREAKFASTS
Ladies and Gentlemen,
Start Your Engines

IT DOESN'T MATTER WHAT KIND of race we're talking about—the Olympic 100-meter dash, the Daytona 500, or the Kentucky Derby—the winner is the person, car, or colt that crosses the finish line first. But in every race, finishing strong isn't the only thing that determines whether you go to the podium or back to the training room.

Often, the key to a first-place finish is getting a really strong start.

In auto racing, racers covet the pole position. In marathons, elite runners start front and center. In horse racing, jockeys want the middle gates so they don't have to make up too much ground on the outside or get too boxed in on the inside. Getting into the best possible starting position sets you up to run a good, strong race—and have the power to kick hard to the finish.

And that's really the way dieting works: Starting the day strong increases the chances you'll end the day even stronger.

By eating a breakfast with protein and slow-burning carbohydrates, you'll have more energy than a mosh pit full of coeds, and you'll cruise through the day feeling satisfied, avoiding the harsh ups and downs that force many of us into a midmorning Snickers fix. So put yourself in position to win the abs race, and get into the starting blocks with these 6-minute meals.

Let's Go Bowling: 6-Pack Breakfast Bowls

You don't have to be a college football fan to appreciate a good bowl. In fact, these bowl-only meals give you the two things you most need for fast breakfasts: fast fixing and little mess.

Slush Fun

Powerfoods: 3

1 teaspoon vanilla whey protein powder

1 cup low-fat plain or vanilla yogurt

½ cup high-fiber breakfast cereal, such as Nature's Path Optimum Power

Stir protein powder into yogurt until well blended. Add cereal; stir.
Serves 1
Nutritional information, per serving: 262 calories, 19 g protein, 38 g carbs, 5 g total fat, 3 g saturated fat, 276 mg sodium, 5 g fiber

You Must Be Nuts

Powerfoods: 5

1 packet instant oatmeal (plus low-fat milk per directions)

½ cup low-fat blueberry fruit-on-the-bottom yogurt, such as Stonyfield Farm

1 tablespoon chopped walnuts

Prepare oatmeal according to package directions, using low-fat milk in place of water. Stir in yogurt until well blended. Top with walnuts.

Serves 1

Nutritional information, per serving: 314 calories, 13 g protein, 46 g carbs, 9 g total fat, 2 g saturated fat, 186 mg sodium, 4 g fiber

Mint Condition

Powerfoods: 2

1 cup low-fat plain or vanilla yogurt

½ teaspoon mint (fresh chopped or dried)

1 cup cubed melon mix

Stir yogurt and mint together until well blended, then toss with melon mixture until completely coated.

Serves 1

Nutritional information, per serving: 208 calories, 14 g protein, 30 g carbs, 4 g total fat, 3 g saturated fat, 197 mg sodium, 1 g fiber

The Chocolate Factory

Powerfoods: 4

½ cup reduced-fat ricotta cheese

½ cup low-fat vanilla yogurt

1 teaspoon chocolate whey protein powder

1 tablespoon chocolate syrup

1 tablespoon chopped pecans

Mix cheese, yogurt, protein powder, and syrup until well blended. Stir in nuts.

Serves 1

Nutritional information, per serving: 336 calories, 20 g protein, 36 g carbs, 12 g total fat, 4 g saturated fat, 209 mg sodium, 2 g fiber

The Lite Lumberjack

Powerfoods: 3

1 egg

1 cup frozen roasted potato cubes

1 microwaveable turkey or lite pork sausage patty

1 tablespoon low-fat shredded Cheddar cheese

Crack egg into a small bowl, stir well until yolk and white are well blended, and micro-wave for 2 minutes, 30 seconds. Microwave potatoes and sausage according to package directions. Chop the sausage. Mix potatoes, sausage, and egg, and top with cheese.

Serves 1

Nutritional information, per serving: 296 calories, 20 g protein, 38 g carbs, 8 g total fat, 3 g saturated fat, 555 mg sodium, 4 g fiber

The 'Bama Bowl

Powerfoods: 4

1   packet instant grits

1   teaspoon ground flaxseed

2   strips beef jerky, finely diced

1   tablespoon low-fat shredded Cheddar cheese

Prepare grits according to package directions. Add flaxseed, jerky, and cheese, stirring well to blend.

Serves 1

Nutritional information, per serving: 199 calories, 11 g protein, 26 g carbs, 6 g total fat, 2 g saturated fat, 786 mg sodium, 3 g fiber

Breakfast with Barbie

Powerfoods: 3

1   packet instant grits

4   frozen shrimp, defrosted and chopped

1   tablespoon low-fat shredded Cheddar cheese

1   dollop barbecue sauce

Prepare grits according to package directions. Add shrimp and cheese, stirring well to blend. Top with barbecue sauce.

Serves 1

Nutritional information, per serving: 167 calories, 9 g protein, 31 g carbs, 1 g total fat, 0 g saturated fat, 731 mg sodium, 2 g fiber

Maple Blessings

Powerfoods: 4

1 packet instant oatmeal (plus low-fat milk per directions)

1 microwaveable turkey or lite pork sausage patty

1 teaspoon ground flaxseed

1 teaspoon maple syrup

Prepare oatmeal according to package directions, using low-fat milk in place of water. Microwave sausage according to package directions. Stir flaxseed and syrup into oatmeal until well blended. Add chopped sausage.

Serves 1

Nutritional information, per serving: 245 calories, 18 g protein, 34 g carbs, 5 g total fat, 2 g saturated fat, 512 mg sodium, 4 g fiber

TRUE GRIT

Maybe the only time you've heard the word "grits" was when that red-haired lady on *Alice* put a "kiss my" in front of them, but this southern specialty is one with which you should familiarize yourself. Grits are made from rough-ground cornmeal; and since corn is a grain, grits qualify as a whole grain Powerfood. Each packet contains 1 gram fiber and 2 grams protein.

The Way to Santa Fe

Powerfoods: 3

1 cup cooked microwaveable brown rice, such as Uncle Ben's

⅓ cup black beans, rinsed and drained

1 egg, fried

¼ cup salsa

Mix together microwaved rice and beans (rice will heat beans). Top with egg and salsa.

Serves 1

Nutritional information, per serving: 384 calories, 16 g protein, 58 g carbs, 9 g total fat, 2 g saturated fat, 547 mg sodium, 8 g fiber

The Texas Two-Step

Powerfoods: 5

1 cup cooked microwaveable brown rice, such as Uncle Ben's

⅓ cup red beans

1 teaspoon diced cilantro

1 egg, fried

1 tablespoon shredded low-fat Mexican-blend cheese

Mix together microwaved rice and beans (rice will heat beans), top with cilantro, egg, and cheese.

Serves 1

Nutritional information, per serving: 379 calories, 16 g protein, 55 g carbs, 10 g total fat, 3 g saturated fat, 234 mg sodium, 7 g fiber

The Package Deal: 6-Pack Breakfast Sandwiches

Most of us think of sandwiches as borderline junk food—great, fleshy slabs of meat slathered in mayo and wedged between two slices of bread. But with the right ingredients, this lunchtime favorite can deliver a knuckle sandwich to your weight worries. Packed with eggs, lean meats, and whole grains, a sandwich can give you a healthy hit of protein, vitamins, minerals, and fiber—and be finished within just a few bites.

Raisin the Stakes

Powerfoods: 3

1 whole wheat toaster waffle

2 tablespoons peanut butter

2 tablespoons raisins or Craisins (dried, sweetened cranberries)

Prepare waffle according to package directions. Spread peanut butter on waffle, top with raisins or Craisins, cut in half, and stack.

Serves 1

Nutritional information, per serving: 349 calories, 12 g protein, 33 g carbs, 21 g total fat, 4 g saturated fat, 134 mg sodium, 4 g fiber

ABS FACT

17 Ounces of cold water needed to boost metabolism by 30 percent for 1½ hours after drinking it, according to a German study

The Sinless Sandwich

Powerfoods: 3

1 whole wheat toaster waffle

2 slices Canadian bacon

1 slice low-fat Cheddar cheese

Prepare waffle according to package directions. Place bacon in center, top with cheese, cut in half, and stack.

Serves 1

Nutritional information, per serving: 223 calories, 20 g protein, 15 g carbs, 9 g total fat, 4 g saturated fat, 881 mg sodium, 1 g fiber

Maple Melt

Powerfoods: 2

1 whole wheat toaster waffle

1 microwaveable turkey or lite pork sausage patty, cooked

1 drizzle maple syrup

Prepare waffle according to package directions. Place heated sausage patty in center, drizzle with syrup, cut in half, and stack.

Serves 1

Nutritional information, per serving: 220 calories, 12 g protein, 30 g carbs, 6 g total fat, 2 g saturated fat, 512 mg sodium, 1 g fiber

IF YOU DON'T HAVE 6 MINUTES . . .

THE BEST READY-MADE OPTIONS FOR BREAKFAST SANDWICHES

Baker's Breakfast Cookies: Granted, they're called cookies, but all varieties are made with rolled oats and whole wheat flour, which means they each contain at least 5 grams of filling fiber. Sweeten the deal—and add a Powerfood—by spreading on a spoonful of all-fruit berry jam.

Swanson's Great Starts Egg, Canadian Bacon, and Cheese Sandwich: A lean protein all-star at 12 grams.

Black Forest Breakfast

Powerfoods: 3

- 1 whole wheat toaster waffle
- 1 tablespoon cranberry relish

- 3 slices deli turkey

Prepare waffle according to package directions. Spread cranberry relish on waffle, top with turkey, cut in half, and stack.

Serves 1

Nutritional information, per serving: 225 calories, 20 g protein, 23 g carbs, 6 g total fat, 1 g saturated fat, 902 mg sodium, 1 g fiber

Guac Your World

Powerfoods: 3

1   whole wheat toaster waffle   2   slices deli turkey

½   avocado, sliced, or 2 tablespoons
     ready-made guacamole, like AvoClassic

Prepare waffle according to package directions. Top with avocado or guacamole and turkey, cut in half, and stack.

Serves 1

Nutritional information, per serving (using ½ fresh avocado): 322 calories, 17 g protein, 24 g carbs, 20 g total fat, 3 g saturated fat, 731 mg sodium, 8 g fiber

Nutritional information, per serving (using 2 tablespoons guacamole): 218 calories, 16 g protein, 19 g carbs, 10 g total fat, 2 g saturated fat, 871 mg sodium, 3 g fiber

---

FREQUENTLY ABS QUESTIONS

I FEEL QUEASY WHEN I EAT BREAKFAST, SO I TEND TO AVOID IT. WHAT'S GOING ON?

If eating breakfast makes your gut feel like it's in a blender, try reducing your intake of fatty foods before you go to bed, because the fat can be what makes you feel bloated in the morning. And opt for bananas over acidic foods like oranges or mangoes; the acid can irritate your stomach.

Waffles Rancheros

Powerfoods: 2

1   egg

1   whole wheat toaster waffle

1   tablespoon salsa

Crack egg in a small bowl, stir well until yolk and white are well blended, and microwave for 2 minutes, 30 seconds. Prepare waffle according to package directions. Top with egg and salsa, cut in half, and stack.

Serves 1

Nutritional information, per serving: 183 calories, 10 g protein, 14 g carbs, 9 g total fat, 3 g saturated fat, 263 mg sodium, 1 g fiber

The Swiss-Army Sandwich

Powerfoods: 3

1   egg

1   whole wheat toaster waffle

1   slice low-fat Swiss cheese

Crack egg in a small bowl, stir well until yolk and white are well blended, and microwave for 2 minutes, 30 seconds. Prepare waffle according to package directions. Top with egg and cheese, cut in half, and stack.

Serves 1

Nutritional information, per serving: 218 calories, 15 g protein, 15 g carbs, 10 g total fat, 3 g saturated fat, 402 mg sodium, 1 g fiber

Best o' the Pesto
Powerfoods: 3

1 egg

1 whole wheat toaster waffle

1 tablespoon ready-made pesto, such as Alessi

Crack egg in a small bowl, stir well until yolk and white are well blended, and microwave for 2 minutes, 30 seconds. Prepare waffle according to package directions. Top with egg and pesto, cut in half, and stack.

Serves 1

Nutritional information, per serving (using 1 tablespoon pesto): 258 calories, 12 g protein, 14 g carbs, 17 g total fat, 4 g saturated fat, 334 mg sodium, 1 g fiber

ABS FACT

2

Number of points by which your "bad" LDL cholesterol can increase after 2 weeks of skipping breakfast, according to one study. It appears that when people don't eat in the morning, they can't process the sudden flood of fat that comes later in the day.

—*American Journal of Clinical Nutrition*

Eggs-Cellent Adventures: 6-Pack Instant Omelets

ABS FACT

69

Percentage of men who eat whatever they want

Besides being the ammunition of choice on mischief night, eggs have one other distinct advantage: They're a powerful source of protein that can be cooked in less time than it takes for a man to tie his tie—especially when you make these instant microwave omelets. For each recipe, stir together 2 eggs in a microwave-safe bowl until they're well blended. Then add remaining ingredients. Nuke for 2 minutes, 30 seconds, or until eggs are set in the middle.

Red All Over

Powerfoods: 2

- 2 eggs
- 1 slice deli roast beef, diced
- 1 slice tomato, diced
- 1 tablespoon diced ready-made roasted red pepper

Serves 1

Nutritional information, per serving: 216 calories, 19 g protein, 7 g carbs, 11 g total fat, 3 g saturated fat, 602 mg sodium, 0 g fiber

Green, Eggs, and Ham
Powerfoods: 3

2   eggs

1   slice Canadian bacon, diced

¼   cup asparagus tips

Serves 1

Nutritional information, per serving: 193 calories, 19 g protein, 3 g carbs, 11 g total fat, 4 g saturated fat, 431 mg sodium, 1 g fiber

Muscle Morning
Powerfoods: 4

2   eggs

1   slice smoked deli turkey, diced

1   tablespoon grated reduced-fat smoked mozzarella cheese

⅓   cup torn baby spinach leaves

Serves 1

Nutritional information, per serving: 235 calories, 26 g protein, 4 g carbs, 12 g total fat, 4 g saturated fat, 551 mg sodium, 0 g fiber

A Breakfast to Relish

Powerfoods: 2

2 eggs

1 tablespoon pickle relish, drained

1 tablespoon diced onion

Serves 1

Nutritional information, per serving: 171 calories, 13 g protein, 7 g carbs, 10 g total fat, 3 g saturated fat, 215 mg sodium, 0 g fiber

Change Your Tuna

Powerfoods: 3

2 eggs

2 tablespoons canned tuna, drained

½ green onion, sliced

Serves 1

Nutritional information, per serving: 189 calories, 20 g protein, 2 g carbs, 10 g total fat, 3 g saturated fat, 249 mg sodium, 1 g fiber

Corn to Be Wild

Powerfoods: 2

2 eggs

2 tablespoons frozen corn kernels

1 slice tomato, chopped

1 tablespoon black beans, rinsed

Serves 1

Nutritional information, per serving: 180 calories, 14 g protein, 7 g carbs, 10 g total fat, 3 g saturated fat, 203 mg sodium, 2 g fiber

Which Came First?

Powerfoods: 3

2 eggs

¼ cup diced precooked chicken

1 slice tomato, diced

1 tablespoon grated reduced-fat mozzarella cheese

Serves 1

Nutritional information, per serving: 254 calories, 31 g protein, 2 g carbs, 13 g total fat, 4 g saturated fat, 228 mg sodium, 0 g fiber

Sombrero Ranchero

Powerfoods: 4

2 eggs

¼ cup diced precooked chicken

½ avocado, chopped

½ teaspoon diced fresh cilantro

Serves 1

Nutritional information, per serving: 393 calories, 31 g protein, 9 g carbs, 26 g total fat, 6 g saturated fat, 183 mg sodium, 7 g fiber

Mo' Feta, Mo' Betta

Powerfoods: 3

2 eggs

½ tablespoon feta cheese crumbles

⅓ cup torn baby spinach leaves

1 sprinkle dried oregano

Serves 1

Nutritional information, per serving: 163 calories, 13 g protein, 2 g carbs, 11 g total fat, 4 g saturated fat, 205 mg sodium, 0 g fiber

Roman Holiday

Powerfoods: 4

2 eggs

2 teaspoons ready-made pesto

¼ cup diced precooked chicken

1 tablespoon grated reduced-fat mozzarella cheese

Serves 1

Nutritional information, per serving: 303 calories, 32 g protein, 1 g carbs, 18 g total fat, 5 g saturated fat, 314 mg sodium, 0 g fiber

THE ABS DIET ULTIMATE POWER BREAKFAST

ON SOME SUNDAY MORNINGS, you crave the all-out, big-momma diner breakfast, where you get not only unlimited coffee but unlimited grease, as well. Instead of lining your belly with half a pig's worth of fat, whip up the ultimate power breakfast in the form of this breakfast bowl. It's brimming with eight Powerfoods to give you the nutrients you need—and the weekend taste you crave.

The Ultimate Power Breakfast
Powerfoods: 8

1 egg

1 cup low-fat milk

¾ cup oatmeal

½ cup mixed berries

1 tablespoon chopped pecans or almonds

1 teaspoon vanilla whey protein powder

1 teaspoon ground flaxseed

½ banana, sliced

1 tablespoon plain yogurt

In microwave-safe bowl, mix egg well, then add next 6 ingredients and nuke for 2 minutes. Remove, let cool for a minute or two. Top with sliced banana and yogurt.

Serves 1

Nutritional information, per serving: 590 calories, 30 g protein, 80 g carbs, 17 g total fat, 4 g saturated fat, 193 mg sodium, 12 g fiber

Chapter 5

6-PACK LUNCHES
The Midday Meal for Midsection Perfection

WHETHER YOU WORK in an office or at home, whether your biggest stressors involve your boss or your kids, lunch is make-or-break time. In many ways, I think lunch is more treacherous than a busted-out bridge. That's because many of us use lunch as the midday escape from insanity. We stop off at bread places, we drive thru for our kids, we celebrate a big account over Flintstone-sized steaks. We want to get out of the office or out of our house because of all the stressful things that are happening inside. But instead of using lunch as a time to escape—often with a bag of burgers and a box of onion rings—we have to think of lunch as halftime. It's our chance to focus on the game plan, refuel our engines, and pack power in a meal that will carry us through to the day's end.

Really, this midday meal (that's meal number 3 of 6, after the midmorning snack) needs to be a time for us to perform a real gut check. And how you do it: with sandwiches, salads, smoothies, or leftovers from a Powerfood dinner. Your options are endless, and any meal from any chapter can really serve as your on-the-go, at-the-desk, or post-hoops lunch. I'll give you some traditional lunch options here, but feel free to steal ideas from other chapters. The concept is still the same no matter what you do during your nutritional nooner.

The Best of Bread: 6-Pack Sandwiches

Sandwiches used to be simple—a little bread, some jelly, some peanut butter, and you were out the door. Now, it seems like the sandwiches we order are either piled higher than a cell phone tower or dripping with dressings, nouveau mayo, and other sauces loaded with more fat than a plastic surgeon's trash can. Instead, make your own power meal with these creations that will fill you up without filling you out.

Join the Club

Powerfoods: 5

2	slices whole wheat bread, toasted	1	slice low-fat pepper Jack cheese
2	slices reduced-sodium smoked turkey, such as Healthy Choice	½	avocado, sliced
2	leaves romaine lettuce		

Toast bread, and top with remaining ingredients.

Serves 1

Nutritional information, per serving: 416 calories, 22 g protein, 41 g carbs, 22 g total fat, 5 g saturated fat, 1,148 mg sodium, 11 g fiber

Reuben Reduced

Powerfoods: 5

¼	cup canned sauerkraut, drained	2	slices rye bread
1	tablespoon feta cheese crumbles	2	slices reduced-sodium smoked deli turkey, such as Healthy Choice
1	tablespoon low-fat Thousand Island dressing	1	slice low-fat Swiss cheese

Coat the bottom of a nonstick skillet with cooking spray, and heat over medium heat.

In a small bowl, stir together kraut, feta cheese, and dressing. Spread kraut mixture on one slice of bread. Top with turkey, Swiss cheese, and remaining slice of bread.

Grill for 2 to 3 minutes per side.

Serves 1

Nutritional information, per serving: 335 calories, 23 g protein, 42 g carbs, 9 g total fat, 3 g saturated fat, 1,625 mg sodium, 5 g fiber

Egg Yourself On

Powerfoods: 5

1 egg

2 slices whole wheat bread

2 slices reduced-sodium deli ham, such as Healthy Choice

1 slice low-fat Cheddar cheese

1 slice tomato

2 leaves romaine lettuce

Lightly coat a nonstick skillet with cooking spray, and add egg. Fry to desired doneness.

While egg cooks, toast bread and assemble sandwich, putting lettuce on as the last layer. Top with hot egg and remaining slice of bread.

Serves 1

Nutritional information, per serving: 331 calories, 28 g protein, 30 g carbs, 11 g total fat, 4 g saturated fat, 950 mg sodium, 4 g fiber

Welcome to Monterey, Jack

Powerfoods: 5

1 egg, whisked

2 slices whole wheat bread

1 tablespoon strawberry jam

2 slices reduced-sodium deli ham, such as Healthy Choice

1 slice low-fat Monterey Jack cheese

Pour whisked egg into a plate.

Assemble sandwich, and dip both sides in the egg.

Place sandwich in a nonstick skillet coated with cooking spray and heated to medium heat. Cook 3 minutes per side, or until golden.

Serves 1

Nutritional information, per serving: 434 calories, 27 g protein, 42 g carbs, 18 g total fat, 9 g saturated fat, 967 mg sodium, 4 g fiber

Perfect PITA
(People for the Intelligent Treatment of Abdominals)

Powerfoods: 4

1 tablespoon barbecue sauce	1 cup chopped romaine lettuce
½ cup chopped precooked chicken	2 tablespoons diced cucumber
1 whole wheat pita	1 tablespoon low-fat ranch dressing

Stir together barbecue sauce and chicken. Microwave for 30 seconds or until hot. Stuff into each pita half.

In a bowl, toss lettuce and cucumber with dressing. Stuff into pitas.

Serves 1

Nutritional information, per serving: 421 calories, 40 g protein, 44 g carbs, 10 g total fat, 2 g saturated fat, 734 mg sodium, 6 g fiber

---

IF YOU DON'T HAVE 6 MINUTES . . .

THE BEST READY-MADE OPTIONS FOR SANDWICHES

Lean Pockets Pepperoni Pizza: Same pizza taste you'd get from the delivery guy, but a fraction of the calories.

Jennie-O Turkey Burgers: 19 grams lean, quick-cooking protein. Take them straight from the freezer and slap 'em down on a hot grill pan.

Omega Foods Wild Salmon Burgers: 1 gram heart-healthy omega-3 fatty acids per burger.

ABS FACT

Iceberg lettuce won't wreck your diet, but it won't do you any nutritional favors, either. Romaine has three times more folate, five times more vitamin C, and nearly eight times more beta-carotene than iceberg.

Roll of a Lifetime
Powerfoods: 4

¾ cup diced precooked chicken

2 tablespoons diced onion

2 tablespoons feta cheese crumbles

1 handful romaine lettuce, chopped

1 large whole wheat tortilla

Salsa for dipping

Arrange chicken, onion, cheese, and lettuce down center of tortilla.

Roll tightly, then cut in half.

Place rolls seam side down on a nonstick skillet heated to medium heat. Grill for 2 to 3 minutes per side. Serve with salsa.

Serves 1

Nutritional information, per serving: 397 calories, 56 g protein, 25 g carbs, 10 g total fat, 4 g saturated fat, 493 mg sodium, 3 g fiber

My Small, Thin Greek Breading

Powerfoods: 4

2   slices reduced-fat mozzarella cheese

1   large whole wheat tortilla

½   cup frozen chopped spinach, defrosted and well drained

¾   cup diced precooked chicken

1   small tomato, diced

Salsa for dipping

Layer cheese on top of tortilla, then top with spinach, chicken, and tomato.

Roll tightly, then cut in half.

Place rolls seam side down on a nonstick skillet heated to medium heat. Grill for 2 to 3 minutes per side. Serve with salsa.

Serves 1

Nutritional information, per serving (salsa not included): 476 calories, 65 g protein, 30 g carbs, 12 g total fat, 6 g saturated fat, 983 mg sodium, 5 g fiber

Lettuce Be Lean: 6-Pack Salads

Salads usually fall into one of two extremes. They're either skimpier than a Brazilian bikini—meaning they fail to fill you up, provide nutrients, or leave you anywhere near satisfied—or they have so much potato salad, blue cheese, and bacon bits piled on that you'd be better off taking a bite out of a cow. If you're going to go green for your main meal, make sure you've powered your salads with the right kinds of ingredients.

Crunch Time

Powerfoods: 5

- 3   cups mixed greens
- 2   slices smoked deli turkey slices, chopped
- ½   small Granny Smith apple, chopped
- 2   tablespoons grated carrot
- 1   tablespoon diced pecans

- 1½   tablespoons Craisins (dried, sweetened cranberries)
- 1   tablespoon blue cheese crumbles

For dressing: 1½ teaspoons olive oil; 1 tablespoon balsamic vinegar

Serves 1

Nutritional information, per serving: 296 calories, 15 g protein, 31 g carbs, 15 g total fat, 3 g saturated fat, 590 mg sodium, 7 g fiber

---

IF YOU DON'T HAVE 6 MINUTES . . .

THE BEST READY-MADE OPTION FOR SALAD

EarthBound Farms Organic Single Serve Grab & Go Salad Kits: Salad in a box—literally. My favorite: Mixed Baby Greens with Classic Vinaigrette and Walnuts. Look for them in your grocery's produce section.

The Two Chicks

Powerfoods: 4

3   cups mixed greens

⅓   cup chickpeas, rinsed and drained

½   cup diced precooked chicken

¼   cup diced ready-made roasted red peppers

1   teaspoon ground flaxseed

For dressing: 1½ tablespoons low-fat ranch dressing, such as Hidden Valley

Serves 1

Nutritional information, per serving: 391 calories, 41 g protein, 27 g carbs, 12 g total fat, 2 g saturated fat, 884 mg sodium, 8 g fiber

Cuke and a Smile

Powerfoods: 6

3   cups mixed greens

¾   cup diced precooked chicken

½   pear, cored and diced

½   cup chopped cucumber

1   tablespoon diced walnuts

1   tablespoon feta cheese crumbles

For dressing: 1½ teaspoons olive oil; 1 tablespoon balsamic vinegar

Serves 1

Nutritional information, per serving: 482 calories, 55 g protein, 23 g carbs, 20 g total fat, 4 g saturated fat, 260 mg sodium, 6 g fiber

The Melon Banquet
Powerfoods: 4

3 cups mixed greens

⅓ cup cubed watermelon

½ cup cubed cantaloupe

2 tablespoons grated carrot

1 ounce smoked salmon, chopped

1 tablespoon pine nuts

1 teaspoon chopped mint

For dressing: 1½ teaspoons olive oil;
2 teaspoons balsamic vinegar;
1 teaspoon lemon juice

Serves 1

Nutritional information, per serving: 274 calories, 11 g protein, 20 g carbs, 19 g total fat, 2 g saturated fat, 635 mg sodium, 5 g fiber

Pimp My Shrimp
Powerfoods: 4

3 cups chopped romaine lettuce

5 large frozen shrimp, defrosted (with tails removed)

½ avocado, diced

⅓ cup frozen corn kernels, defrosted

1 cup grape tomatoes

2 tablespoons crushed tortilla chips

1 teaspoon chopped cilantro

For dressing: 1½ tablespoons low-fat ranch dressing, such as Hidden Valley

Serves 1

Nutritional information, per serving: 395 calories, 13 g protein, 38 g carbs, 24 g total fat, 4 g saturated fat, 439 mg sodium, 14 g fiber

Mesquite Bites

Powerfoods: 7

3 cups chopped romaine lettuce

¾ cup diced mesquite-flavored precooked chicken

⅓ cup kidney beans, rinsed and drained

½ avocado, diced

2 tablespoons sliced green onions

1 teaspoon chopped cilantro

For dressing: 1½ teaspoons olive oil; 1 tablespoon red wine vinegar; 1 dash paprika

Serves 1

Nutritional information, per serving: 490 calories, 44 g protein, 28 g carbs, 24 g total fat, 3 g saturated fat, 1,276 mg sodium, 14 g fiber

THE 6-PACK QUIZ

Which of these dishes has the most calories?

a. Typical chicken Caesar salad

b. Burger King Whopper

c. Medium-size movie theater popcorn

a. Caesar salad contains over 1,800 calories—1,000 more than a Whopper.

Popeye and Olive Oil

Powerfoods: 4

1½   cups chopped baby spinach leaves

1½   cups chopped romaine lettuce

3   slices prosciutto, chopped

⅓   cup mandarin orange slices

⅓   cup sliced strawberries

2   tablespoons diced red onion

For dressing: 1½ teaspoons olive oil;
   1 tablespoon red wine vinegar;
   ½ clove garlic, crushed;
   ⅛ teaspoon black pepper

Serves 1

Nutritional information, per serving: 238 calories, 9 g protein, 23 g carbs, 14 g total fat, 4 g saturated fat, 450 mg sodium, 6 g fiber

Caesar the Great

Powerfoods: 5

3   cups chopped romaine lettuce

¾   cup diced precooked chicken

1   cup grape tomatoes

¼   cup chopped pitted black or kalamata olives

3   teaspoons grated Parmesan cheese

For dressing: 3 anchovy fillets, diced; 3 teaspoons olive oil; ½ clove garlic, crushed; ⅛ teaspoon black pepper

Serves 1

Nutritional information, per serving: 520 calories, 58 g protein, 14 g carbs, 26 g total fat, 5 g saturated fat, 938 mg sodium, 7 g fiber

Olive a Good Tuna

Powerfoods: 4

2	(3–4 ounces each) fresh yellowfin or ahi tuna fillets	¼	cup roughly chopped roasted red pepper (thumbnail-size pieces)
5	cups chopped romaine lettuce		For dressing: 2 tablespoons olive oil; 2 tablespoons lemon juice; 1 tablespoon grainy Dijon mustard; ¼ teaspoon dried thyme; 1 clove garlic, crushed
1¾	cups grape tomatoes		
⅓	cup whole pitted black or kalamata olives		

Sear tuna in a nonstick skillet heated over medium-high heat (no more than 1 minute per side). Season each side with a pinch of salt and pepper as it cooks. Remove tuna from skillet and set aside.

In a large bowl, stir together lettuce, tomatoes, olives, and pepper.

In a small bowl, stir together dressing ingredients until well blended.

Cut tuna into ½" thick slices. Divide salad mixture between two plates, and top with tuna and dressing.

Serves 2

Nutritional information, per serving: 631 calories, 50 g protein, 34 g carbs, 35 g total fat, 5 g saturated fat, 1,123 mg sodium, 11 g fiber

DRIVE-THRU CREATIONS

Between tight schedules and on-the-road meetings, eating fast food is sometimes as unavoidable as catching a glimpse of Andy Dick on TV. Here are some options for turning a weak moment into a strong one.

THE ORDER	THE PLAN
Plain grilled chicken sandwich 1 cup of chili	Add the protein you need, dump the carbs you don't. Toss the bun. Pour chili on top of chicken, and top with torn lettuce and cut-up tomato from the sandwich.
Plain grilled chicken sandwich Baked potato with sour cream	Make a more nutritious "sandwich." Eat the potato and sour cream, leaving the skin. Toss the empty-calorie bun, and put the chicken inside the potato skin (that's where all the potato's nutrients are). Top with salsa and eat like a sandwich.
Small vanilla shake Fruit and yogurt parfait	Supersize your order without supersizing your gut. Dump half the shake into another cup. Add yogurt and fruit and stir well to blend. Eat with a spoon.

Chapter 6

6-PACK DINNERS
The Dinners That Will Make You Thinner

THERE'S AN OLD SAYING among fitness circles: Eat breakfast like a king, lunch like a prince, and dinner like a pauper. It sounds like a smart philosophy—until you realize that in today's America, paupers eat at KFC.

In fact, it's the thrifty and resourceful among us who can control their weight by controlling their stress and controlling their food intake. And perhaps the hardest meal of all to control is dinner. So often it's not in our hands—it's whatever's on the menu, or what the take-out place has to offer, or what Mom's whipping up for dinner because "you know you never come to visit and it's so nice to see my baby. . . . "

Dinner can be a celebration of a good day's work, a time to socialize with friends and family, a time to sit back, enjoy, and wait patiently until your prime-time pundit of choice starts his show. I'm all for unwinding, socializing, and celebrating a job well done, but I think we make a mistake when we put all our calories in one basket.

What you need to do is treat your dinner like any other meal—pump it up with Powerfoods, and let it satisfy you without sabotaging you. I can tell you that once people start getting used to eating four times before they even have dinner, their appetites are significantly reduced—meaning that your body eventually gets it. It gets that you don't need to gorge at dinner. It gets that you don't have to make the last big meal of the day worthy of being the last meal of your life.

Create Quite a Stir: 6-Pack Stir-Fries

You don't have to be named O'Reilly or Matthews to enjoy stirring things up. One of my favorite kinds of Powerfood dinners is a good stir-fry. Dump your Powerfoods into a skillet, cook them quickly, and you wind up with a dish that has more flavors than Cold Stone Creamery.

The Bell Ringer

Powerfoods: 3

- 2 teaspoons peanut oil
- ¼ teaspoon red pepper flakes
- 2 thin-cut boneless, skinless chicken breasts, cut into bite-size pieces or strips
- 1 cup green or red bell pepper, cut into bite-size pieces or strips
- ¼ medium onion, cut into bite-size pieces or strips
- 2 teaspoons reduced-sodium soy sauce

Combine oil and pepper flakes in a medium-hot skillet.

Add chicken and cook for 2 to 3 minutes, stirring frequently.

Add remaining ingredients and cook for 2 to 3 minutes, stirring frequently. Serve over brown rice.

Serves 1

Nutritional information, per serving: 320 calories, 42 g protein, 12 g carbs, 11 g total fat, 2 g saturated fat, 472 mg sodium, 3 g fiber

TIME FOR AN OIL CHANGE

Ordinarily, I recommend olive oil (after all, it's the O in Abs Diet Power). But because it can burn when you use it to cook foods at high temperatures, switch to peanut oil for stir-fries. Since it's made from Powerfood-worthy nuts, peanut oil still counts as an abs-friendly food.

The Orange and Gold

Powerfoods: 5

2 teaspoons peanut oil	⅓ cup chopped celery
¼ teaspoon red pepper flakes	1 green onion, sliced
2 thin-cut boneless, skinless chicken breasts, cut into bite-size pieces or strips	2 tablespoons chopped unsalted roasted peanuts
⅓ cup matchstick carrots	1 tablespoon hoisin sauce

Combine oil and pepper flakes in a medium-hot skillet.

Add chicken and cook for 2 to 3 minutes, stirring frequently.

Add remaining ingredients and cook for 2 to 3 minutes, stirring frequently. Serve over brown rice.

Serves 1

Nutritional information, per serving: 356 calories, 45 g protein, 18 g carbs, 11 g total fat, 2 g saturated fat, 444 mg sodium, 5 g fiber

The Almond Brothers

Powerfoods: 5

2 teaspoons peanut oil

¼ teaspoon red pepper flakes

2 thin-cut boneless, skinless chicken breasts, cut into bite-size pieces or strips

½ cup asparagus tips

⅓ cup matchstick carrots

¼ medium onion, cut into bite-size pieces or strips

⅓ cup frozen snow peas

2 tablespoons sliced almonds

2 teaspoons reduced-sodium soy sauce

Combine oil and pepper flakes in a medium-hot skillet.

Add chicken and cook for 2 to 3 minutes, stirring frequently.

Add remaining ingredients and cook for 2 to 3 minutes, stirring frequently. Serve over brown rice.

Serves 1

Nutritional information, per serving: 428 calories, 48 g protein, 20 g carbs, 18 g total fat, 3 g saturated fat, 505 mg sodium, 7 g fiber

Clockwork Orange
Powerfoods: 3

2	teaspoons peanut oil	½	cup frozen snow peas
¼	teaspoon red pepper flakes	2	teaspoons orange juice
2	thin-cut pork chops, cut into bite-size pieces or strips	2	teaspoons reduced-sodium soy sauce
¼	medium onion, cut into bite-size pieces or strips	¼	teaspoon orange zest

Combine oil and pepper flakes in a medium-hot skillet.

Add pork and cook for 2 to 3 minutes, stirring frequently.

Add remaining ingredients and cook for 2 to 3 minutes, stirring frequently. Serve over brown rice.

Serves 1

Nutritional information, per serving: 410 calories, 41 g protein, 14 g carbs, 21 g total fat, 6 g saturated fat, 438 mg sodium, 3 g fiber

ABS FACT

600
Number of calories by which people underestimate the size of their restaurant meals

Chop Chop!

Powerfoods: 3

- 2 teaspoons peanut oil
- ¼ teaspoon red pepper flakes
- 2 thin-cut pork chops, cut into bite-size pieces or strips
- 1 small zucchini, cut into bite-size pieces or strips
- ⅓ medium onion, cut into bite-size pieces or strips
- ⅓ cup matchstick carrots
- 1 clove garlic, crushed
- 2 teaspoons reduced-sodium soy sauce

Combine oil and pepper flakes in a medium-hot skillet.

Add pork and cook for 2 to 3 minutes, stirring frequently.

Add remaining ingredients and cook for 2 to 3 minutes, stirring frequently. Serve over brown rice.

Serves 1

Nutritional information, per serving: 406 calories, 40 g protein, 15 g carbs, 21 g total fat, 6 g saturated fat, 473 mg sodium, 3 g fiber

The Loin King

Powerfoods: 4

2 teaspoons peanut oil	2 teaspoons reduced-sodium soy sauce
¼ teaspoon red pepper flakes	1 teaspoon honey
1 cup thinly sliced sirloin strips	1 clove garlic, crushed
½ cup frozen snow peas	¼ teaspoon lemon zest
½ cup chopped celery	
2 teaspoons lemon juice	

Combine oil and pepper flakes in a medium-hot skillet.

Add sirloin and cook for 2 to 3 minutes, stirring frequently.

Add remaining ingredients and cook for 2 to 3 minutes, stirring frequently. Serve over brown rice.

Serves 1

Nutritional information, per serving: 492 calories, 47 g protein, 18 g carbs, 25 g total fat, 8 g saturated fat, 501 mg sodium, 4 g fiber

The Broc Heads

Powerfoods: 5

2   teaspoons peanut oil

¼   teaspoon red pepper flakes

1   cup thinly sliced sirloin strips

1   cup chopped broccoli (bite-size pieces)

¼   medium onion, chopped into bite-size pieces or strips

¼   cup chopped green bell pepper (bite-size pieces or strips)

1   egg, whisked

2   teaspoons reduced-sodium soy sauce

Combine oil and pepper flakes in a medium-hot skillet.

Add sirloin and cook for 2 to 3 minutes, stirring frequently.

Add remaining ingredients and cook for 2 to 3 minutes, stirring frequently. Serve over brown rice.

Serves 1

Nutritional information, per serving: 532 calories, 53 g protein, 11 g carbs, 30 g total fat, 9 g saturated fat, 540 mg sodium, 3 g fiber

Veggin' Out

Powerfoods: 6

2 teaspoons peanut oil

¼ teaspoon red pepper flakes

¼ medium onion, chopped into bite-size pieces or strips

⅓ cup frozen snow peas

⅓ cup matchstick carrots

⅓ cup chopped broccoli (bite-size pieces)

¼ cup chopped green or red bell pepper (bite-size pieces or strips)

1 egg, whisked

1 tablespoon hoisin sauce

1 teaspoon reduced-sodium soy sauce

1 cup black beans, rinsed and drained

Combine oil and pepper flakes in a medium-hot skillet.

Add everything but the beans (they'll burn and become tough if you cook them too long). Cook for 2 to 3 minutes, stirring frequently.

Add beans and cook for another 2 to 3 minutes, stirring frequently. Serve over brown rice.

Serves 2

Nutritional information, per serving: 285 calories, 15 g protein, 35 g carbs, 9 g total fat, 2 g saturated fat, 819 mg sodium, 12 g fiber

Shrimp to Nuts

Powerfoods: 4

2   teaspoons peanut oil

¼   teaspoon red pepper flakes

½   cup French green beans, cut into bite-size pieces

⅓   cup matchstick carrots

¼   cup whole unsalted roasted cashews

2   teaspoons reduced-sodium soy sauce

2   teaspoons orange juice

¼   teaspoon orange zest

1½   cups medium frozen shrimp, defrosted with tails removed

Combine oil and pepper flakes in a medium-hot skillet.

Add everything but the shrimp (they're already precooked before freezing). Cook for 2 to 3 minutes, stirring frequently.

Add shrimp and cook for another 2 to 3 minutes, stirring frequently. Serve over brown rice.

Serves 2

Nutritional information, per serving: 332 calories, 39 g protein, 11 g carbs, 15 g total fat, 3 g saturated fat, 578 mg sodium, 2 g fiber

ABS FACT

20

Number of minutes it takes your stomach to realize it's full

Pepper Prawns

Powerfoods: 4

2 teaspoons peanut oil

¼ teaspoon red pepper flakes

1 cup chopped green or red bell pepper (bite-size pieces or strips)

¼ medium onion, cut into bite-size pieces or strips

2 tablespoons canned jalapeño chile pepper slices

1 tablespoon orange juice

1 tablespoon hoisin sauce

1½ cups medium frozen shrimp, defrosted with tails removed

Combine oil and pepper flakes in a medium-hot skillet.

Add everything but the shrimp (they're already precooked before freezing). Cook for 2 to 3 minutes, stirring frequently.

Add shrimp and cook for another 2 to 3 minutes, stirring frequently. Serve over brown rice.

Serves 2

Nutritional information, per serving: 256 calories, 37 g protein, 10 g carbs, 7 g total fat, 1 g saturated fat, 594 mg sodium, 2 g fiber

Major Meals: 6-Pack Meat and Vegetable Meals

Growing up, many of us knew exactly what we'd have for dinner: a hunk of meat, a side of vegetables, and something with more starch than a Wall Streeter's dress shirt. There's nothing wrong with craving the good ole dinner days. Just make that starch brown rice or whole wheat pasta, and add these meat and vegetable combos.

Gone Fishing

Powerfoods: 5

1 tablespoon + 1 teaspoon olive oil	½ teaspoon chopped fresh parsley
1 trout fillet	1 cup French green beans, trimmed and cut into bite-size pieces
1 tablespoon cornmeal	
Salt and pepper to taste	2 teaspoons sliced almonds

Heat 1 tablespoon oil in a nonstick skillet over medium heat.

While pan is heating, sprinkle flesh side of trout with cornmeal, salt, and pepper, pressing lightly so the cornmeal sticks.

Place in pan, flesh side down, and sauté for 4 minutes. Flip and cook for another 2 minutes. Top with parsley.

Place beans into a steamer basket and steam for 5 minutes. Toss with remaining 1 teaspoon oil, almonds, salt, and pepper.

Serves 1

Nutritional information, per serving: 372 calories, 20 g protein, 17 g carbs, 26 g total fat, 4 g saturated fat, 48 mg sodium, 5 g fiber

Slammin' Salmon
Powerfoods: 6

1	can (7 ounces) pink salmon, drained	¼	teaspoon red pepper flakes
1	egg, whisked	2	tablespoons peanut oil
½	cup crushed whole wheat crackers	4	cups mixed greens
2	tablespoons diced green onion	2	tablespoons low-fat ranch dressing
1	teaspoon Old Bay seasoning		

In a large bowl, mix together salmon, egg, crackers, onion, Old Bay, and red pepper flakes.

Form into 2 large patties or 4 small ones.

Add oil to a nonstick skillet heated to medium.

Place patties in pan and sauté 3 minutes on each side, or until golden. Drain on a paper towel.

For salad, toss greens and dressing in a large bowl to coat. Divide between two plates, and top with salmon patties.

Serves 2

Nutritional information, per serving: 448 calories, 22 g protein, 23 g carbs, 31 g total fat, 6 g saturated fat, 763 mg sodium, 5 g fiber

Here's Your Cue

Powerfoods: 3

2 teaspoons olive oil	2 tablespoons barbecue sauce
1 clove garlic, crushed	1 thick slice of onion
1½ cups thinly sliced sirloin	

Combine oil and garlic in a nonstick skillet over medium-high heat.

Add sirloin and cook 2 to 3 minutes, until browned.

Reduce heat to low, and add barbecue sauce, stirring well to coat.

Lightly brush onion with olive oil, then lay it on a grill pan heated to medium-high heat. Cook for 6 minutes, turning once.

Serves 2

Nutritional information, per serving: 312 calories, 33 g protein, 6 g carbs, 16 g total fat, 5 g saturated fat, 228 mg sodium, 0 g fiber

---

IF YOU DON'T HAVE 6 MINUTES . . .

THE BEST READY-MADE OPTIONS FOR MEAT AND VEGETABLE DINNERS

Healthy Choice Beef Merlot: Red wine makes this meal heated in a microwave taste like it's not.

Smart Ones Stuffed Turkey Breast: Thanksgiving in a box.

Lean Cuisine Salmon with Basil: This one's packed with Powerfoods: salmon, peppers, and whole wheat pasta.

An Apple Today

Powerfoods: 2

2   teaspoons olive oil

1   small clove garlic, crushed

2   thin-cut boneless pork chops

1   small soft red apple, such as Gala or Red Delicious, cored and diced

2   teaspoons balsamic or red wine vinegar

1   tablespoon bourbon

1   tablespoon grainy mustard

Salt and pepper to taste

Combine oil and garlic in a nonstick skillet over medium-high heat.

Add pork chops to center of skillet. Toss apple with vinegar and bourbon, then add apple mixture to the skillet between the pork and the edges of the pan.

Cook for 6 minutes, turning pork once and turning apple pieces a few times.

When ready to serve, top pork with mustard. Season to taste with salt and pepper.

Serves 1

Nutritional information, per serving: 459 calories, 38 g protein, 17 g carbs, 21 g total fat, 5 g saturated fat, 401 mg sodium, 4 g fiber

Colonel Mustard

Powerfoods: 3

1 tablespoon maple syrup

1 tablespoon Dijon mustard

1 teaspoon olive oil

Salt and pepper to taste

2 thin-cut boneless pork chops

2 cups Italian salad greens

1 tablespoon low-fat balsamic vinaigrette

In a small bowl, stir together syrup, mustard, oil, salt, and pepper until well blended.

Place chops and mustard mixture inside a large zip-top plastic bag, then shake to coat the chops.

Place chops on a nonstick skillet heated to medium-high, cooking 2 to 3 minutes per side. In last minute of cooking, pour remaining mustard mixture onto chops as they cook.

Toss greens and dressing in a large bowl to coat.

Serves 1

Nutritional information, per serving: 393 calories, 42 g protein, 23 g carbs, 17 g total fat, 5 g saturated fat, 650 mg sodium, 2 g fiber

THE THIN COMMANDMENTS

The thinner the meat, the faster it will cook—and that's a crucial element when you're trying to prepare a meal in fewer than 6 minutes. These recipes call for thin-cut pork and chicken, which you can find easily at your grocery store's meat counter. Thin cuts of beef are a little harder to find, but you can make your own. Just slip your cut into the freezer for a few minutes to firm it up, then slice away!

Chicken Little Italy

Powerfoods: 3

1 tablespoon + 1 teaspoon olive oil	Salt and pepper to taste
1 boneless, skinless chicken breast	¼ cup marinara sauce
1 tablespoon Italian-seasoned bread crumbs	1 small clove garlic, crushed
1 teaspoon Parmesan cheese	3 handfuls baby spinach leaves

Heat 1 tablespoon oil in a nonstick skillet over medium heat.

While pan is heating, pound chicken to ¼" thickness, then sprinkle with bread crumbs, cheese, salt, and pepper, pressing lightly so crumbs stick.

Place in pan and sauté for 2 to 3 minutes per side. Top with nuked marinara.

Combine remaining 1 teaspoon oil and garlic in another nonstick skillet over medium-high heat.

Add spinach, turning frequently with tongs until wilted (about 6 minutes).

Serves 1

Nutritional information, per serving: 395 calories, 32 g protein, 19 g carbs, 22 g total fat, 3 g saturated fat, 608 mg sodium, 5 g fiber

We've Got to Stop Meating Like This: 6-Pack Vegetarian Meals

Depending on where you stand on the whole cow issue—or more important, where the person you're dating stands on it—you can still follow the Abs Diet with Powerfoods substitutions. Instead of lean meats and fish, you can sub in soy (in the form of tofu) and beans for many main-meat dishes. Or try the following vegetarian-friendly options.

Mr. Green Beans
Powerfoods: 4

1   teaspoon olive oil

1   clove garlic, crushed

¼   teaspoon red pepper flakes

4   cups chopped kale

1   cup white beans, rinsed and drained

2   tablespoons pine nuts

⅓   cup beer

Heat oil, garlic, and pepper flakes in a large skillet over medium-high heat. Add kale, beans, nuts, and beer. Cover and cook for 6 minutes, turning occasionally with tongs until liquid evaporates.

Serves 2

Nutritional information, per serving: 256 calories, 12 g protein, 33 g carbs, 12 g total fat, 2 g saturated fat, 399 mg sodium, 9 g fiber

Egg-Drop, Pounds-Drop Soup
Powerfoods: 2

4	eggs	1	quart vegetable stock
½	teaspoon black pepper	2	green onions, sliced
¼	teaspoon red pepper flakes		

Whisk together eggs, pepper, and pepper flakes. Pour the egg mixture slowly into a pot of boiling stock, stirring with a whisk. Remove from stove, and stir continually until eggs form ribbons—about 1 minute. Before serving, drop in green onions.

Serves 2

Nutritional information, per serving: 229 calories, 15 g protein, 15 g carbs, 11 g total fat, 3 g saturated fat, 980 mg sodium, 4 g fiber

Tofu You Too!

Powerfoods: 6

2   teaspoons peanut oil

1   cup frozen extra-firm tofu, defrosted and cut into bite-size pieces

2   teaspoons rice vinegar

1   tablespoon hoisin sauce

½   cup black beans, rinsed and drained

1   green onion, sliced

2   tablespoons sliced almonds

2   cups cooked microwaveable brown rice, such as Uncle Ben's

Heat oil in a nonstick skillet over medium-high heat.

Add tofu and cook for 2 to 3 minutes, turning occasionally.

Add vinegar, hoisin sauce, beans, green onion, and almonds, stirring occasionally. Serve over rice.

Serves 2

Nutritional information, per serving: 449 calories, 21 g protein, 59 g carbs, 15 g total fat, 2 g saturated fat, 293 mg sodium, 9 g fiber

HOW TO HANDLE TOFU

As soon as you bring a block of extra-firm tofu home from the store, pop it into the freezer, where it can stay for up to a month. Freezing changes the tofu's texture—it'll turn brown and kind of chewy. In other words, it becomes a lot more like meat.

Jump for Soy

Powerfoods: 2

2	teaspoons peanut oil	1	tablespoon reduced-sodium soy sauce
¼	teaspoon red pepper flakes		
6	slices frozen extra-firm tofu, defrosted		

Combine oil and pepper flakes in a nonstick skillet over medium-high heat.

Add tofu and soy sauce, and cook for 2 to 3 minutes, turning occasionally.

Serves 2

Nutritional information, per serving: 270 calories, 25 g protein, 3 g carbs, 20 g total fat, 3 g saturated fat, 292 mg sodium, 3 g fiber

---

IF YOU DON'T HAVE 6 MINUTES . . .

THE BEST READY-MADE OPTIONS FOR VEGETARIAN DINNERS

Healthy Choice Stuffed Pasta Shells: Three big cheese-stuffed shells in tangy tomato sauce make this microwave dinner feel like a meal.

Seeds of Change Seven Grain Pilaf Microwaveable Bowl: Better than most brands' beef or chicken options, and better for you, too. The wholesome mix of whole grains is made slightly less so by lots of cheese.

Progresso 99% Fat-Free Minestrone: A good source of lean protein and fiber, thanks to the kidney beans. Slap together a grilled low-fat cheese on whole wheat, and you have a great weeknight meal.

Twice the Spice

Powerfoods: 6

1 tablespoon olive oil

¼ teaspoon red pepper flakes

1 cup frozen extra-firm tofu, defrosted and cut into bite-size pieces

½ cup diced red bell pepper

¼ cup diced unsalted cashews

¼ cup diced matchstick carrots

2 cloves garlic, crushed

2 tablespoons diced canned jalapeño chile peppers

2 teaspoons reduced-sodium soy sauce

1 green onion, sliced

5 iceberg lettuce leaves, washed and dried

Combine oil and red pepper flakes in a nonstick skillet over medium heat. Add tofu and cook, turning occasionally, for 2 to 3 minutes.

Add remaining ingredients except for lettuce leaves, stirring well to blend. Cook for 2 to 3 minutes, while continually stirring. Serve with lettuce leaves.

Serves 2

Nutritional information, per serving: 315 calories, 17 g protein, 16 g carbs, 22 g total fat, 4 g saturated fat, 654 mg sodium, 5 g fiber

Eggs Insalata

Powerfoods: 4

2 eggs, whisked	2 cups Italian salad mix
⅓ cup white beans, rinsed and drained	1 tablespoon low-fat Italian dressing
2 tablespoons feta cheese crumbles	Salt and pepper to taste
⅛ teaspoon rosemary	

In a large bowl, mix whisked eggs, beans, cheese, and rosemary. Pour into a nonstick skillet over medium heat, and cook for 6 minutes, stirring occasionally to raise cooked eggs from bottom of pan. While eggs cook, mix greens and dressing in a bowl, tossing to coat. Serve eggs on top of greens. Season with salt and pepper to taste.

Serves 1

Nutritional information, per serving: 299 calories, 22 g protein, 19 g carbs, 17 g total fat, 6 g saturated fat, 918 mg sodium, 7 g fiber

ABS FACT

64 Percentage of Americans who don't believe obese people are to blame for their weight

Shroom, Shroom, Shroom!

Powerfoods: 2

1 teaspoon olive oil

2 large portobello mushroom caps,
   wiped clean

2 slices low-fat Swiss cheese

Heat olive oil in nonstick skillet over medium-high heat. Place mushrooms in skillet top side down. Cook for 3 minutes. Flip mushrooms, and add 1 slice cheese to each. Cook for another 3 minutes.

Serves 1

Nutritional information, per serving: 211 calories, 17 g protein, 19 g carbs, 7 g total fat, 2 g saturated fat, 419 mg sodium, 4 g fiber

Romaines of the Day
Powerfoods: 5

2	cups chopped romaine lettuce hearts	1	tablespoon diced fresh cilantro
1	medium avocado, chopped into bite-size pieces	1	tablespoon olive oil
1	medium tomato, chopped into bite-size pieces	2	teaspoons lime juice
½	cup black beans, rinsed and drained	¼	teaspoon lime zest
2	tablespoons diced green onion	¼	teaspoon salt
		½	teaspoon pepper

Toss lettuce, avocado, tomato, beans, green onion, and cilantro together in a large bowl.

In a small bowl, stir together oil, lime juice, zest, salt, and pepper. Pour over salad, and toss well to coat.

Serves 2

Nutritional information, per serving: 295 calories, 6 g protein, 24 g carbs, 22 g total fat, 3 g saturated fat, 436 mg sodium, 11 g fiber

Have a Whole Pie: 6-Pack Pizzas

It used to be that pizza was diet death—between the greasy cheese, the shred-ded sausage, the perfectly paunch-forming pepperoni, and the thick, chewy crust, it was a veritable coronary delivered to your door in 30 minutes or less. But that doesn't have to be the case—if you know how to take advantage of its good ingredients (tomato sauce, whole wheat crusts, vegetables, and lean meats).

License to Kielbasa

Powerfoods: 3

- 3 tablespoons reduced-fat ricotta cheese
- 1 ready-made flatbread, such as Flat Out
- ¾ cup thinly sliced turkey kielbasa
- ¼ cup diced onion
- 3 tablespoons grated reduced-fat mozzarella cheese

Spread ricotta on flatbread. Top with kielbasa, onion, and mozzarella. Bake at 375°F for 6 minutes.

Serves 1

Nutritional information, per serving: 414 calories, 34 g protein, 40 g carbs, 13 g total fat, 7 g saturated fat, 1,796 mg sodium, 3 g fiber

Terra Ricotta

Powerfoods: 3

- 3 tablespoons reduced-fat ricotta cheese
- 1 teaspoon ready-made roasted garlic
- 1 ready-made flatbread, such as Flat Out
- ¾ cup chopped precooked chicken
- 3 tablespoons grated reduced-fat mozzarella cheese
- Salt and pepper to taste

Stir together ricotta and garlic, blending well. Spread on flatbread. Top with chicken and mozzarella. Season to taste with salt and pepper. Bake at 375°F for 6 minutes.

Serves 1

Nutritional information, per serving: 352 calories, 41 g protein, 19 g carbs, 13 g total fat, 6 g saturated fat, 409 mg sodium, 2 g fiber

IF YOU DON'T HAVE 6 MINUTES . . .

THE BEST READY-MADE OPTION FOR PIZZA

Stouffer's French Bread Pizzas: These crunchy single-serving pizzas are light-years better than delivery, especially because you won't have the leftovers tempting you during your 3 a.m. infomercial marathon.

Green Daze

Powerfoods: 3

3   tablespoons reduced-fat ricotta cheese

1   teaspoon ready-made roasted garlic

1   ready-made flatbread, such as Flat Out

1   tablespoon ready-made pesto

2   tablespoons ready-made roasted red peppers

3   tablespoons grated reduced-fat mozzarella cheese

Salt and pepper to taste

Stir together ricotta and garlic, blending well. Spread on flatbread. Top with dollops of pesto, peppers, and mozzarella. Season to taste with salt and pepper. Bake at 375°F for 6 minutes.

Serves 1

Nutritional information, per serving: 306 calories, 15 g protein, 25 g carbs, 16 g total fat, 6 g saturated fat, 768 mg sodium, 2 g fiber

Spinach City
Powerfoods: 5

3 tablespoons reduced-fat ricotta cheese	¼ cup diced onion
1 ready-made flatbread, such as Flat Out	¾ cup chopped precooked chicken
⅓ cup frozen spinach, defrosted and thoroughly drained	3 tablespoons grated reduced-fat mozzarella cheese
1 tablespoon ready-made pesto	Salt and pepper to taste

Spread ricotta on flatbread. Stir together spinach and pesto, blending well. Spread on flatbread. Top with onion, chicken, and mozzarella. Season to taste with salt and pepper. Bake at 375°F for 6 minutes.

Serves 1

Nutritional information, per serving: 564 calories, 63 g protein, 26 g carbs, 24 g total fat, 8 g saturated fat, 655 mg sodium, 5 g fiber

---

PESTO CHANGE-O!

You might have to hunt for ready-made pesto in the average grocery store (look for little jars of the stuff near the pasta and other Italian foods), but the Italian sauce is one of the smartest condiments you can purchase. It's basically a blend of three Power-foods—olive oil, leafy green basil and spinach, and pine nuts, with some Parmesan cheese tossed in, too. Yes, it's fatty, but all the fats in pesto are good ones, courtesy of the oil and nuts. The same can't be said for ranch dressing, mayo, or Alfredo sauces, which are mostly saturated fat. Use pesto in place of them as a dip, on sandwiches or pizzas, or mixed with a little vinegar as a flavor-packed salad dressing.

The Greek God

Powerfoods: 4

3   tablespoons marinara sauce

1   ready-made flatbread, such as Flat Out

⅓   cup frozen spinach, defrosted and thoroughly drained

¼   cup feta cheese crumbles

¾   cup chopped precooked chicken

1   tablespoon sliced fresh basil

Salt and pepper to taste

Spread marinara on flatbread. Top with spinach, feta, chicken, and basil. Season to taste with salt and pepper. Bake at 375°F for 6 minutes.

Serves 1

Nutritional information, per serving: 533 calories, 62 g protein, 24 g carbs, 21 g total fat, 10 g saturated fat, 1,020 mg sodium, 4 g fiber

Heavenly Honolulu

Powerfoods: 2

3	tablespoons marinara sauce	1	teaspoon red pepper flakes
1	ready-made flatbread, such as Flat Out	3	tablespoons grated low-fat Cheddar cheese
3	slices deli ham, chopped		Salt and pepper to taste
2½	tablespoons crushed pineapple, thoroughly drained		

Spread marinara on flatbread. Top with ham, pineapple, pepper flakes, and Cheddar. Season to taste with salt and pepper. Bake at 375°F for 6 minutes.

Serves 1

Nutritional information, per serving: 255 calories, 22 g protein, 27 g carbs, 6 g total fat, 2 g saturated fat, 1,090 mg sodium, 4 g fiber

Thai It, You'll Like It

Powerfoods: 5

3 tablespoons peanut butter

2 teaspoons soy sauce

1 ready-made flatbread, such as Flat Out

2 tablespoons sliced green onions

¾ cup chopped and defrosted frozen shrimp

1 tablespoon sliced fresh basil

3 tablespoons grated reduced-fat mozzarella cheese

Stir together peanut butter and soy sauce, blending well. Spread on flatbread. Top with onions, shrimp, basil, and mozzarella. Bake at 375°F for 6 minutes.

Serves 1

Nutritional information, per serving: 599 calories, 56 g protein, 27 g carbs, 31 g total fat, 7 g saturated fat, 1,033 mg sodium, 6 g fiber

BBQ Za
Powerfoods: 3

¼   cup barbecue sauce

1   ready-made flatbread, such as Flat Out

¼   cup canned diced tomatoes with chiles and onions or garlic, well drained

¾   cup precooked mesquite-flavor chicken

2   tablespoons sliced green onions

1   teaspoon diced cilantro

3   tablespoons grated reduced-fat mozzarella cheese

Spread barbecue sauce on flatbread. Top with tomatoes, chicken, onions, cilantro, and mozzarella. Bake at 375°F for 6 minutes.

Serves 1

Nutritional information, per serving: 411 calories, 39 g protein, 41 g carbs, 10 g total fat, 4 g saturated fat, 1,059 mg sodium, 3 g fiber

Chapter 7

6-PACK SNACKS, SMOOTHIES, AND SAUCES

IN THEIR WORST FORMS, side dishes, snacks, and sauces can drape hundreds of extra calories onto any meal. You can negate the low-fat goodness of a chicken breast by dripping melted full-fat cheese and bacon all over it. You can spoil a perfectly good potato with full-fat sour cream. And you can cancel out your whole wheat pasta if you order it with a topping of sausage. While they make up part of the nutritional supporting cast, sauces and side dishes can steal the show the way Kramer used to steal diner scenes in *Seinfeld*—they add a doofus note to an otherwise perfectly sane meal. Sides and condiments should push your taste buds to the limits, but they shouldn't do the same for your seams.

In this miscellaneous chapter, you'll find foods you can make to go with main dishes, add as dipping sauces for vegetables, or even whip up as desserts. Whatever the case, they're the kinds of sides you want on your side.

Shake It Up: 6-Pack Smoothies

When you adopt the Abs Diet, your blender should work out harder than Jack LaLanne. Smoothies are the easiest—and one of the best—possible meals you can make. Dump a few ingredients, push a button, then swig. In this book, the smoothie recipes take more of a dessert twist to satisfy your late-night or post-dinner sweet cravings. For more breakfast- and lunch-type smoothies, please see *The Abs Diet* and *The Abs Diet Eat Right Every Time Guide*.

Belly-Busting Berry
Powerfoods: 6

1   scoop low-fat vanilla ice cream

¼   cup each frozen blueberries, strawberries, and raspberries

½   cup low-fat milk

1   tablespoon vanilla whey protein powder

3   ice cubes

Serves 1

Nutritional information, per smoothie: 251 calories, 15 g protein, 38 g carbs, 4 g total fat, 2 g saturated fat, 116 mg sodium, 4 g fiber

Coco Poof

Powerfoods: 4

1 scoop low-fat chocolate ice cream	½ banana
½ cup frozen raspberries	3 ice cubes
½ cup low-fat chocolate milk	
1 tablespoon chocolate whey protein powder	

Serves 1

Nutritional information, per smoothie: 340 calories, 17 g protein, 56 g carbs, 7 g total fat, 4 g saturated fat, 145 mg sodium, 6 g fiber

Strawberry Shortcut

Powerfoods: 4

1 scoop low-fat strawberry ice cream	1 tablespoon vanilla whey protein powder
½ cup frozen strawberries	3 ice cubes
½ banana	
½ cup low-fat milk	

Serves 1

Nutritional information, per smoothie: 283 calories, 14 g protein, 48 g carbs, 4 g total fat, 2 g saturated fat, 106 mg sodium, 5 g fiber

Extreme Chocolate

Powerfoods: 3

1	scoop low-fat chocolate ice cream	½	banana
1	tablespoon chocolate syrup	3	ice cubes
½	cup low-fat chocolate milk		
1	tablespoon chocolate whey protein powder		

Serves 1

Nutritional information, per smoothie: 355 calories, 17 g protein, 60 g carbs, 6 g total fat, 4 g saturated fat, 158 mg sodium, 4 g fiber

Pumpkin You Up!

Powerfoods: 3

1	scoop low-fat butter pecan ice cream	1	teaspoon ground flaxseed
½	cup canned pumpkin	3	ice cubes
½	cup low-fat milk		
1	tablespoon vanilla whey protein powder		

Serves 1

Nutritional information, per smoothie: 265 calories, 17 g protein, 41 g carbs, 5 g total fat, 2 g saturated fat, 136 mg sodium, 7 g fiber

Blue Cheesecake

Powerfoods: 6

1 scoop low-fat vanilla ice cream

½ cup reduced-fat ricotta cheese

½ cup low-fat milk

1 tablespoon vanilla whey protein powder

2 tablespoons low-fat plain yogurt

½ cup frozen blueberries

3 ice cubes

Serves 1

Nutritional information, per smoothie: 400 calories, 28 g protein, 44 g carbs, 14 g total fat, 8 g saturated fat, 307 mg sodium, 3 g fiber

Dark Vader

Powerfoods: 4

1 scoop low-fat chocolate ice cream

½ cup reduced-fat ricotta cheese

½ cup low-fat chocolate milk

1 tablespoon chocolate whey protein powder

1 teaspoon ground flaxseed

3 ice cubes

Serves 1

Nutritional information, per smoothie: 400 calories, 29 g protein, 40 g carbs, 15 g total fat, 10 g saturated fat, 315 mg sodium, 2 g fiber

Lemon Drips and Drops

Powerfoods: 5

1	scoop low-fat vanilla ice cream	1	tablespoon sliced almonds
½	cup reduced-fat ricotta cheese	½	lemon, juiced and zested
½	cup low-fat milk	3	ice cubes
1	tablespoon vanilla whey protein powder		

Serves 1

Nutritional information, per smoothie: 387 calories, 27 g protein, 37 g carbs, 16 g total fat, 8 g saturated fat, 289 mg sodium, 2 g fiber

Show Me the Honey

Powerfoods: 3

1	scoop low-fat butter pecan ice cream	1	dash cinnamon
½	cup low-fat milk	1	teaspoon honey
1	tablespoon vanilla whey protein powder	3	ice cubes
1	teaspoon ground flaxseed		

Serves 1

Nutritional information, per smoothie: 250 calories, 15 g protein, 38 g carbs, 4 g total fat, 2 g saturated fat, 131 mg sodium, 3 g fiber

Okay on the OJ

Powerfoods: 4

1 scoop low-fat orange sherbet

½ cup peeled, ready-to-eat cantaloupe

½ cup reduced-fat ricotta cheese

½ cup low-fat milk

½ cup orange juice

1 tablespoon vanilla whey protein powder

3 ice cubes

Serves 1

Nutritional information, per serving: 438 calories, 25 g protein, 60 g carbs, 12 g total fat, 8 g saturated fat, 290 mg sodium, 1 g fiber

ABS FACT

3 Number of daily kiwifruit that will reduce your risk of heart attack. Best tactic: Drop one or two in your smoothie.

Let's Choose Up Sides: 6-Pack Side Dishes

Side dishes are like dentists' instructions—they get ignored a lot. But instead of treating side dishes like floss, why not supercharge your meal with these Powerfood-rich offerings—some of which can accompany a meal or even stand on their own?

A Good Game of Squash

Powerfoods: 1

2	zucchini	1	tablespoon Parmesan cheese
2	yellow summer squash		Salt and pepper to taste

Slice zucchini and squash into rounds. Arrange in steamer and steam for 3 to 5 minutes. Remove, pat dry with paper towel, and toss with cheese. Season to taste with salt and pepper.

Serves 2

Nutritional information, per serving: 58 calories, 5 g protein, 10 g carbs, 1 g total fat, 0 g saturated fat, 68 mg sodium, 3 g fiber

Turbo Tomatoes

Powerfoods: 1

2   large beefsteak tomatoes

2   teaspoons olive oil

1   teaspoon balsamic vinegar

Salt and pepper to taste

Slice tomatoes into ½"-thick rounds (each tomato should yield 3 to 4 slices).

Drizzle with oil and vinegar. Season to taste with salt and pepper.

Place on baking sheet lightly coated with cooking spray. Broil for 3 to 4 minutes.

Serves 2

Nutritional information, per serving: 59 calories, 2 g protein, 9 g carbs, 3 g total fat, 0 g saturated fat, 17 mg sodium, 2 g fiber

---

IF YOU DON'T HAVE 6 MINUTES . . .

THE BEST READY-MADE OPTIONS FOR SIDE DISHES

Bush's Original Microwaveable Cup: One of the best ready-made sides, period. These baked beans provide enough protein and fiber (11 grams each) for a meal.

Uncle Ben's Ready Rice, Brown: This microwaveable brown rice cooks in its own packet, so you don't even have to dirty a pot.

Vigo Red Beans and Rice: Less salty than most ready-made rice and bean mixes, with 7 grams of protein and 4 grams of fiber.

Birds Eye Pepper Stir-Fry Mix: Antioxidants? They're in the bag. And once this blend of peppers is nuked in the microwave, you'd never know they were frozen in the first place.

Sweet, Sour, and Simple Salad

Powerfoods: 2

1   head endive

1   small green apple

1   tablespoon diced walnuts

1   tablespoon low-fat balsamic vinaigrette

Peel off outer leaves of endive (think of it as a single-serving head of lettuce), and chop into bite-size pieces. Chop apple, removing core. Toss well, then top with nuts and dressing.

Serves 1

Nutritional information, per serving: 226 calories, 8 g protein, 43 g carbs, 7 g total fat, 1 g saturated fat, 297 mg sodium, 21 g fiber

See Slaw

Powerfoods: 3

2 cups packaged broccoli slaw	2 tablespoons chopped almonds
⅓ cup diced onion	2 teaspoons sesame oil
½ cup grated carrot	1½ tablespoons rice wine vinegar
1 tablespoon diced fresh cilantro	¼ teaspoon red pepper flakes

In a large bowl, mix together slaw, onion, carrot, cilantro, and almonds.

In a small bowl, stir together oil, vinegar, and pepper flakes. Pour over vegetable mixture, tossing well to coat.

Serves 1

Nutritional information, per serving: 291 calories, 11 g protein, 30 g carbs, 16 g total fat, 2 g saturated fat, 95 mg sodium, 6 g fiber

Serves 2

Nutritional information, per serving: 146 calories, 6 g protein, 15 g carbs, 8 g total fat, 1 g saturated fat, 48 mg sodium, 3 g fiber

Veg-Infused Couscous

Powerfoods: 3

½	cup couscous	1	tablespoon chopped almonds
½	yellow squash, diced	½	teaspoon mint
½	red bell pepper, diced	½	teaspoon olive oil
1	tablespoon feta cheese crumbles		Salt and pepper to taste

Prepare couscous according to package directions.

Add remaining ingredients and toss well to blend.

Serves 2

Nutritional information, per serving: 210 calories, 8 g protein, 38 g carbs, 3 g total fat, 1 g saturated fat, 62 mg sodium, 4 g fiber

No-Sufferin' Succotash

Powerfoods: 3

1 cup frozen baby lima beans

1 cup frozen corn kernels

½ small onion, diced

1 clove garlic, crushed

½ red bell pepper, diced

1 teaspoon olive oil

⅓ cup low-fat shredded Cheddar cheese

Salt and pepper to taste

Place frozen beans and corn in colander, and run hot water over them until defrosted. Drain well.

Sauté onion, garlic, and bell pepper in oil in nonstick pan over medium heat (about 4 minutes).

Add beans-and-corn mixture and cheese, stirring well to blend. Season to taste with salt and pepper.

Serves 2

Nutritional information, per serving: 256 calories, 14 g protein, 41 g carbs, 5 g total fat, 1 g saturated fat, 275 mg sodium, 9 g fiber

Take It from the Top: 6-Pack Sauces and Salsas

Alfredo and queso sauces aren't the only sauces that will fatten you up. Some sauces, toppings, and dips can turn your carrots into carnage, your squash into squish, your lima beans into lardo beans. You're safe with olive oil and vinegar—as well as these quick-whipped dips.

Dill-icious Dip
Powerfoods: 3

1	cup low-fat plain yogurt	¼	cup diced onion
⅓	cup diced cucumber	½	teaspoon dill

Stir ingredients together in a small bowl until well blended.

Nutritional information, per 1-tablespoon serving: 10 calories, 1 g protein, 1 g carbs, 0 g total fat, 0 g saturated fat, 9 mg sodium, 0 g fiber

---

THE FIX IS IN

IF YOU NEED . . .	GRAB . . .
Something salty, crunchy	Dill spears (1 calorie each) will cover both cravings.
To decide on a restaurant side	Vegetables instead of rice will decrease calories and keeps insulin levels low.
To use up your Starbucks gift card	Use fat-free milk and avoid drinks with mocha, toffee, or chai in the name. On average, you'll cut calorie content by 75 percent.

Sweet on Salsa

Powerfoods: 2

1	mango, diced	2	teaspoons chopped cilantro
¼	cup diced red bell pepper	½	teaspoon red pepper flakes
¼	cup diced onion		Salt and pepper to taste
1	tablespoon olive oil		

Stir ingredients together in a small bowl until well blended.

Nutritional information, per 1-tablespoon serving: 18 calories, 0 g protein, 3 g carbs, 1 g total fat, 0 g saturated fat, 0 mg sodium, 0 g fiber

Honey-Nut Mustard

Powerfoods: 2

1	cup Dijon mustard	2	tablespoons diced pecans
¼	cup honey	2	teaspoons olive oil

In blender or food processor, mix mustard, honey, and nuts. Stream oil through the top until you reach desired consistency (aim for kind of thick but spreadable if you want to use it on sandwiches).

Nutritional information, per 1-tablespoon serving: 28 calories, 2 g protein, 5 g carbs, 1 g total fat, 0 g saturated fat, 240 mg sodium, 0 g fiber

Rip-Roarin' Roasted Red-Pepper Sauce

Powerfoods: 3

1 jar (7 ounces) ready-made roasted red peppers, drained and chopped

2 tablespoons chopped fresh basil

2 tablespoons diced walnuts

1 clove garlic, crushed

1 teaspoon balsamic vinegar

1 tablespoon olive oil

Salt and pepper to taste

In blender or food processor, mix peppers, basil, nuts, garlic, and vinegar. Stream oil through the top until you reach desired consistency. Season to taste with salt and pepper.

Nutritional information, per 1-tablespoon serving: 23 calories, 0 g protein, 1 g carbs, 2 g total fat, 0 g saturated fat, 45 mg sodium, 0 g fiber

ABS FACT

If you need to hit the vending machine, hit the numbers for the candy bar that best fits our Powerfood profile: Payday. It has 260 calories and 12 grams of unsaturated fat—but only 2 grams of saturated fat. (Mounds, for example, has 10 grams of the saturated stuff.)

Spread Yourself Thin

Powerfoods: 2

1 can (15 ounces) cannellini beans, rinsed and drained

1 tablespoon chopped fresh rosemary

1 clove garlic, crushed

½ lemon, juiced

2 tablespoons olive oil

Salt and pepper to taste

In blender or food processor, mix beans, rosemary, garlic, and lemon juice. (If you're using a blender, you may need to stop and scrape the sides of the canister once to make sure everything blends well.) Stream oil through the top until you reach desired consistency. Season to taste with salt and pepper.

Nutritional information, per 1-tablespoon serving: 21 calories, 1 g protein, 2 g carbs, 1 g total fat, 0 g saturated fat, 20 mg sodium, 1 g fiber

The Tweeners: 6-Pack Snacks

Growing up, our snacks fit into three major food groups: exploded popcorn, deep-fried potato chips, and whatever it is that eventually becomes a Dorito. Now, our snacks can consist of any Powerfood combo—peanut butter on whole grain, a handful of nuts and chocolate milk, or a bowl of berries and yogurt. Or concoct one of these.

Berry Up to the Bar

Powerfoods: 2

- 2 tablespoons blueberries
- 1 peanut butter–flavored Clif Bar

Crush blueberries in a small bowl with a fork. Spread crushed blueberries onto the flat side of the Clif Bar.

Serves 1

Nutritional information, per serving: 250 calories, 12 g protein, 41 g carbs, 5 g total fat, 1 g saturated fat, 289 mg sodium, 5 g fiber

---

ABS FACT

70 Number of almonds eaten daily by people who dropped 18 percent of their body weight in a 6-month study

PB Power Apples

Powerfoods: 2

2 tablespoons peanut butter

1 dash cinnamon

1 medium red apple, such as Gala or Red Delicious, halved and cored

In a small bowl, stir together peanut butter and cinnamon (start with a dash—cinnamon is potent stuff). Spread peanut butter mixture on each apple half.

Serves 1

Nutritional information, per serving: 276 calories, 8 g protein, 30 g carbs, 17 g total fat, 3 g saturated fat, 1 mg sodium, 8 g fiber

Master Lox Smith

Powerfoods: 3

4 green onions, sliced

1 packet (8 ounces) smoked salmon, chopped

½ teaspoon pepper

8 ounces low-fat cream cheese, softened

Stir onions, salmon, and pepper into softened cream cheese until well mixed. Eat with whole wheat crackers or celery.

Serves 40

Nutritional information, per 1-teaspoon serving: 21 calories, 2 g protein, 1 g carbs, 1 g total fat, 1 g saturated fat, 131 mg sodium, 0 g fiber

Screamin' Creamin' Veggies

Powerfoods: 3

¼ cup ready-made roasted red peppers, drained and diced

¼ cup diced cucumber

2 tablespoons diced fresh parsley

½ teaspoon pepper

8 ounces low-fat cream cheese, softened

Stir red peppers, cucumber, parsley, and pepper into softened cream cheese until well mixed. Eat with whole wheat crackers or celery.

Serves 30

Nutritional information, per 1-teaspoon serving: 28 calories, 1 g protein, 1 g carbs, 2 g total fat, 1 g saturated fat, 48 mg sodium, 0 g fiber

---

IF YOU DON'T HAVE 6 MINUTES . . .

THE BEST READY-MADE OPTIONS FOR SNACKS

Blue Diamond Smoked Almonds: Awesome smokehouse flavor and less sodium than even some reduced-sodium brands.

Smart Balance Light Butter Popcorn: Balances "light" with "butter" perfectly. Plus, no nasty hydrogenated oils.

Snyder's of Hanover Carb Fix Pretzel Sticks: Won't chip your teeth, like so many other pretzels. Plus, 9 grams of belly-filling fiber per serving.

Kashi Trail Mix Bars: Packed with nuts and sweetened only with natural sugars. Plus, 4 grams of fiber per bar make this a snack that'll stay with you.

PACK YOUR SNACKS

SNACKS UNDER 200 CALORIES	SNACKS UNDER 400 CALORIES
Stick of string cheese (80)	One egg on whole grain English muffin with melted cheese (250)
Skippy brand squeeze stick of peanut butter (140)	Clif bar (250)
5 cups light microwave popcorn sprinkled with hot sauce and/or 1 tablespoon of Romano cheese (150)	Peanut butter and jelly on whole grain English muffin (300)
6 strawberries dipped in yogurt, drizzled with chocolate sauce (150)	Oatmeal with milk; add brown sugar, walnuts, and any fresh or dried fruit (300)
Canned tuna with balsamic vinegar on whole grain crackers (175)	Slice of whole grain bread topped with peanut butter and banana (300)
1 cup reduced-sodium cottage cheese with fresh peaches and cinnamon (200)	½ cup hummus with roasted vegetables (400)
Two handfuls of olives (200)	
1 cup blackberries, blueberries, or strawberries with 6 ounces of light yogurt and 1 tablespoon of low-fat granola (200)	

Cucumber Tubes

Powerfoods: 5

1 medium-size cucumber	½ teaspoon finely chopped chives
1 teaspoon finely chopped parsley	¾ cup low-fat, low-sodium cottage cheese
¼ teaspoon finely chopped basil	

Cut cucumber in half lengthwise. Hollow the center of each cucumber half by scooping out seeds with a spoon or vegetable knife. Stir finely chopped herbs into cottage cheese, then arrange in hollowed cucumbers.

Serves 2

Nutritional information, per serving: 84 calories, 12 g protein, 7 g carbs, 1 g total fat, 1 g saturated fat, 11 mg sodium, 2 g fiber

FREQUENTLY ABS QUESTION

GRANOLA BARS: YAY OR NAY?

Don't make them a regular snack: Besides being high in calories, they have another effect: Every time you eat a bar that contains high amounts of sugar (that's most of them), your blood-glucose level rises quickly. In turn, this stimulates the release of insulin, which signals your body to store fat. Best to make your own mixture of nuts, dry granola, and dried fruit.

The Finish Line: 6-Pack Desserts

If you pummeled your innards with pantry-stored or bakery-made desserts, you'd undoubtedly wind up with a belly large enough to house a family of four. But to deny yourself all sweets isn't the answer—especially when you can make these after-dinner indulgences.

Berried Alive

Powerfoods: 5

1 cup each frozen blueberries, strawberries, and raspberries

¼ cup balsamic vinegar

1 teaspoon dried basil

Sprinkle of sugar

1 scoop reduced-fat ice cream, such as Edy's Grand Light

Place berries, vinegar, basil, and sugar in a plastic container. Shake well to mix, then store in the fridge (should last for up to a week). Top a scoop of your favorite reduced-fat ice cream with ½ cup of berry mixture.

Serves 6

Nutritional information, per serving: 262 calories, 6 g protein, 43 g carbs, 8 g total fat, 5 g saturated fat, 84 mg sodium, 3 g fiber

Bananacicles

Powerfoods: 1

4	Popsicle sticks
2	bananas, peeled and cut in half crosswise
½	cup chocolate sauce (the kind that forms a shell)
4	tablespoons unsalted peanuts, diced

Put a Popsicle stick into the cut end of each banana piece. Pour chocolate sauce over bananas until they're completely coated. Roll chocolate-coated bananas in peanuts. Freeze.

Serves 4

Nutritional information, per serving: 318 calories, 4 g protein, 32 g carbs, 22 g total fat, 9 g saturated fat, 21 mg sodium, 4 g fiber

Yogi Pops

Powerfoods: 1

1 6-pack (4-ounce cups) of your favorite
   flavor of reduced-fat yogurt

6 Popsicle sticks

Pierce each yogurt pack with a stick. Freeze.

Serves 6

Nutritional information, per serving: 118 calories, 4 g protein, 24 g carbs, 1 g total fat, 0 g saturated fat, 59 mg sodium, 0 g fiber

IF YOU DON'T HAVE 6 MINUTES . . .

THE BEST READY-MADE OPTIONS FOR DESSERTS

Edy's Grand Light Ice Cream: Most Edy's Grand Light flavors have only a couple of grams of saturated fat, compared to double-digit counts in traditional ice cream.

Cold Fusion Ice Cream Bars: They're made with at least 10 grams of muscle-building whey protein.

Snickers Almond Candy Bar: Healthy unsaturated fat courtesy of the almonds, plus a creamy, gooey center.

Barbara's Whole-Wheat Fig Bars: The nutty whole grain casing makes these bars taste even sweeter than ordinary ones. Plus, 1 gram of fiber.

Pepperidge Farm Soft Baked Oatmeal Raisin Cookies: Big, man-size cookies contain 2 grams of fiber, thanks to their Powerfood-packed ingredients.

Your Sundae Best

Powerfoods: 2

1   crunchy granola bar, such as Nature
    Valley Peanut Butter

1   scoop reduced-fat vanilla ice cream

2   teaspoons maple syrup

Crumble granola bar on top of ice cream. Top with syrup.

Serves 1

Nutritional information, per serving: 267 calories, 7 g protein, 38 g carbs, 11 g total fat, 5 g saturated fat, 156 mg sodium, 1 g fiber

Piece of Cake

Powerfoods: 2

2   slices ready-made frozen pound cake

2   teaspoons chocolate hazelnut spread
    (such as Nutella)

3   strawberries, sliced

Slice cake and place on a medium-hot grill pan. Grill for 1 to 2 minutes per side. Spread with chocolate and berries, then top with another slice of cake, like a sandwich.

Serves 2

Nutritional information, per serving: 340 calories, 6 g protein, 46 g carbs, 15 g total fat, 7 g saturated fat, 283 mg sodium, 2 g fiber

BONUS SECTION

6-PACK EXTRAS
More Time, More Options

THE WHOLE REASON I created the 6-minute meals in this book is because I know that you don't have time to spend in the kitchen day after day, flipping this, waiting for that. But I also like to think that there are some days when you might not be in such a rush—and you can use that to your 6-minute advantage. For example, there are plenty of 60-minute and 15-minute Powerfood meals that you can make to eat right then and there or to save to heat up throughout the week. The advantage: Investing a little more time equals more options and more tastes.

60 Minutes: 6-Pack Sunday Creations

Let's just assume you can take an hour between games or playing with your kids to make a perfect weekend meal—or one that you can reuse during the week as a premade lunch or heat-it-right-up dinner.

Mexi-Peppers
Powerfoods: 4

½   pound 90% lean ground beef

4   ounces low-fat refried beans

¾   cup salsa (drain extra liquid)

1   ounce dark chocolate, chopped

½   teaspoon cumin

6   large jalapeño chile peppers, cut in half lengthwise, seeds removed

12   tablespoons low-fat shredded Cheddar cheese

Brown beef in a nonstick skillet over medium-high heat. Once cooked, drain fat.

Add beans, salsa, chocolate, and cumin to beef, stirring well to blend. (If you like spicy food, save the jalapeño pepper seeds, and stir them into the ground beef mixture.)

Once beef mixture has cooled, spoon it into the chile peppers and top each with 1 tablespoon cheese.

Bake at 325°F for 15 to 20 minutes.

Or freeze individual servings (2 peppers) in zip-top plastic bags. To reheat, bake peppers on a pan at 375°F for 20 to 25 minutes.

Serves 3

Nutritional information, per serving: 286 calories, 25 g protein, 16 g carbs, 13 g total fat, 6 g saturated fat, 549 mg sodium, 4 g fiber

Stew for You

Powerfoods: 1

1   pound sirloin steak, cubed

1   onion, chopped

2   cloves garlic, crushed

3   carrots, chopped

2   cups white mushrooms

2   cups frozen roasted potato cubes

1   teaspoon pepper

½   teaspoon salt

2   cans (10.5 ounces each) low-fat beef broth

1   tablespoon flour

1   cup red wine

Brown beef in a nonstick skillet over medium-high heat (about 2 to 3 minutes). Once cooked, drain fat and set aside beef.

In same skillet, sauté onion, garlic, carrots, mushrooms, and potatoes until soft (about 6 minutes).

In a large stock pot, mix beef, sautéed vegetables, pepper, and salt, stirring well to blend.

In a small bowl, whisk together beef broth, flour, and wine. Pour broth mixture over beef and vegetable mixture, stirring well to blend. Simmer over medium-low heat for 30 minutes, adding additional broth or wine if needed.

To reheat, microwave for 2 to 3 minutes, stirring once.

Serves 6

Nutritional information, per serving: 231 calories, 21 g protein, 22 g carbs, 4 g total fat, 1 g saturated fat, 671 mg sodium, 3 g fiber

The Monster Meat Mash
Powerfoods: 2

1	pound 90% lean ground beef	½	cup low-fat beef broth
1	small onion, diced	6	cups prepared mashed potatoes
2	cloves garlic, crushed	1	cup low-fat shredded Cheddar cheese
½	cup barbecue sauce		
2	teaspoons flour		

Brown beef in a nonstick skillet over medium-high heat. Once cooked, drain fat and set aside beef.

In same skillet, sauté onion and garlic until soft (about 6 minutes).

In a casserole dish, mix beef, onion, and barbecue sauce, stirring well to blend.

In a separate small bowl, whisk together flour and beef broth. Pour broth mixture over beef mixture. Top with potatoes and cheese.

Bake at 350°F for 30 minutes.

To reheat, microwave for 2 to 3 minutes, stirring once.

Serves 6

Nutritional information, per serving: 401 calories, 26 g protein, 47 g carbs, 12 g total fat, 5 g saturated fat, 931 mg sodium, 0 g fiber

Souped Up

Powerfoods: 4

2   carrots, chopped

1   large onion, chopped

4   zucchini or yellow squash, chopped

3   cloves garlic, crushed

1   tablespoon olive oil

3   cans (16 ounces) low-sodium chicken broth

1   can (15 ounces) white beans, rinsed and drained

1   can (14 ounces) diced Italian-seasoned tomatoes

½   teaspoon salt

½   teaspoon pepper

1   teaspoon oregano

2   cups spinach

In large stock pot, sauté carrots, onion, zucchini or squash, and garlic in oil until soft (about 6 minutes).

Add broth, beans, tomatoes, salt, pepper, and oregano. Stir well, reduce heat to low, and simmer for 30 minutes to an hour. Just before you're ready to eat, stir in spinach and let it wilt (about 2 minutes).

Serves 6

Nutritional information, per serving: 165 calories, 12 g protein, 27 g carbs, 4 g total fat, 1 g saturated fat, 679 mg sodium, 7 g fiber

Chicken Soup for the Bowl

Powerfoods: 4

1	rotisserie chicken	½	teaspoon thyme
4	stalks celery, diced	½	teaspoon salt
2	carrots, diced	½	teaspoon pepper
1	onion, diced	⅔	cup uncooked brown rice
2	cloves garlic, crushed	3	cans (16 ounces each) low-sodium chicken broth (optional)
2	teaspoons olive oil		

Slice breasts off chicken, dice, wrap, and refrigerate. Tear apart the rest of the chicken, and place pieces in a large stock pot, covered with water. Bring to a boil, then simmer for 1 hour.

Place a colander in a large bowl and strain chicken liquid. Remove chicken parts, tearing off any meat. Set aside stock and meat.

In cleaned pot, sauté celery, carrots, onion, and garlic in oil until soft (about 6 minutes).

Add chicken meat (including refrigerated breast meat), stock, thyme, salt, pepper, and rice. Bring to a boil, then simmer for 30 minutes, adding water or low-sodium chicken broth if needed.

Serves 6

Nutritional information, per serving: 251 calories, 22 g protein, 26 g carbs, 7 g total fat, 2 g saturated fat, 356 mg sodium, 3 g fiber

It's a Little Chili in Here

Powerfoods: 2

1 pound 90% lean ground beef	½ teaspoon salt
1 onion, diced	½ teaspoon pepper
3 cloves garlic, crushed	1 teaspoon chili powder
2 cans (15 ounces each) kidney beans, rinsed and drained	½ teaspoon cumin
	⅛ teaspoon cayenne
2 cans (8 ounces each) no-salt-added diced tomatoes	⅛ teaspoon cinnamon
	1 ounce dark chocolate, chopped
2 cans (10.75 ounces each) low-sodium chicken broth	

Brown beef in a nonstick skillet over medium-high heat. Once cooked, drain most of the fat and set aside.

In same skillet, sauté onion and garlic until soft in a little bit of remaining beef fat (about 6 minutes).

In a large stock pot, add cooked beef, onion and garlic, beans, tomatoes, broth, spices, and chocolate. Simmer on low heat for 1 hour.

Serves 6

Nutritional information, per serving: 311 calories, 26 g protein, 29 g carbs, 10 g total fat, 4 g saturated fat, 631 mg sodium, 7 g fiber

Anytime, Anywhere, Anyplace Pasta Sauce

Powerfoods: 2

1	pound ground turkey breast	1	can (16 ounces) diced tomatoes
1	small onion, diced	1	teaspoon basil
3	cloves garlic, crushed	½	teaspoon salt
3	ounces canned tomato paste	½	teaspoon pepper

Brown turkey in a nonstick skillet over medium-high heat. Once cooked, drain most of the fat and set aside.

In same skillet, sauté onion and garlic until soft in a little bit of remaining turkey fat (about 6 minutes).

Place cooked turkey, onion, and garlic in a large stock pot. Add paste, tomatoes, basil, salt, and pepper. Simmer over medium-low heat for 30 minutes.

Serving size: 1 cup

Nutritional information, per serving: 236 calories, 41 g protein, 17 g carbs, 2 g total fat, 0 g saturated fat, 906 mg sodium, 2 g fiber

ANY-WHICH-WAY CHICKEN

Spend 30 minutes making chicken breasts on Sunday, and you can have lean protein for lunch or dinner all week. Add diced cold chicken to salads or make sandwiches or entrées with the whole breasts by zapping them in the microwave. To boost the flavor, marinate them with one of the choices below.

- 1 tablespoon ready-made Italian dressing per breast
- 1 tablespoon bourbon, 1 teaspoon grainy mustard per breast
- 1 teaspoon lemon juice, ⅛ teaspoon powdered garlic, and ⅛ teaspoon thyme per breast
- 2 teaspoons balsamic vinegar, 1 teaspoon olive oil, ⅛ teaspoon rosemary per breast
- 1 teaspoon hot sauce, 1 teaspoon honey, 1 teaspoon orange juice per breast
- 1 tablespoon low-fat yogurt, ⅛ teaspoon dill per breast
- 1 teaspoon low-sodium soy sauce, 2 teaspoons pineapple juice, 1 dash cayenne pepper per breast
- 2 teaspoons red wine, 1 teaspoon barbecue sauce, ⅛ teaspoon garlic powder per breast

Mix marinade ingredients in a zip-top plastic bag. Add chicken and let it marinate for 30 minutes. Drop marinated breasts onto a hot grill pan and sear for 2 to 3 minutes per side. Let them cool, then place in individual zip-top bags and refrigerate for up to 5 days.

Speed Up the Action: 6-Pack 15-Minute Meals

If you're not rushing off to late meetings, soccer practice, or your friend's weekly *Extreme Makeover* social, then you should have the prep time to make these 15-minute meals.

Beast of the East

Powerfoods: 3

½ pound sirloin, sliced diagonally into thin strips

1 cup seeded and chopped green or red bell pepper (thumbnail-size pieces)

1 cup chopped onion (thumbnail-size pieces)

2 tablespoons reduced-sodium soy sauce

1 teaspoon sugar

1½ teaspoons olive oil

1 clove garlic, crushed

1 teaspoon red pepper flakes

Dump all ingredients into a large zip-top plastic bag. Shake and set aside for 1 minute or 1 hour.

Pour meat, sauce, and vegetables into a medium-hot cast-iron skillet, and cook, stirring frequently, until meat is seared and vegetables begin to lose water (about 2 to 3 minutes).

Serves 2

Nutritional information, per serving: 253 calories, 28 g protein, 17 g carbs, 8 g total fat, 2 g saturated fat, 601 mg sodium, 3 g fiber

Thai One On

Powerfoods: 4

1	tablespoon extra-virgin olive oil	1	can (14 ounces) reduced-sodium beef broth
⅓	pound 90% lean sirloin steak, diced	⅓	cup creamy peanut butter
½	package McCormick beef-stew seasoning mix		
16	ounces frozen mixed vegetables		

Heat the oil in a large, heavy pot. Add the steak and cook over medium-high heat until well browned.

Add the seasoning mix, and stir in the vegetables.

Turn heat to high. Add the beef broth; bring to a boil.

Reduce heat to medium-high, and stir in the peanut butter.

Serves 4

Nutritional information, per serving: 291 calories, 17 g protein, 20 g carbs, 16 g total fat, 3 g saturated fat, 810 mg sodium, 5 g fiber

Not-So-Sloppy Joes

Powerfoods: 2

⅓ pound 90% lean ground beef

1 clove garlic, crushed

⅓ cup low-sodium barbecue sauce

1 can small refrigerator biscuits (5)

Salt and pepper to taste

½ cup low-fat shredded Cheddar cheese

Brown beef in a nonstick skillet over medium heat until well browned.

Add garlic and barbecue sauce; stir well and sauté for 1 minute more.

While beef is browning, mash biscuits into a nonstick muffin tin, forming cups. Place hot beef mixture into cups. Season to taste with salt and pepper. Top with cheese, then bake according to biscuit package directions for 8 to 10 minutes.

Serves 2

Nutritional information, per serving: 536 calories, 28 g protein, 49 g carbs, 25 g total fat, 7 g saturated fat, 1,202 mg sodium, 3 g fiber

Red and Blue Salad
Powerfoods: 2

9   ounces flank steak

Salt and pepper to taste

2   plum tomatoes, cut into eighths

⅓   cup vertically sliced onion

1   small clove garlic, crushed

5   cups chopped romaine lettuce

4   tablespoons low-fat balsamic vinaigrette

3   tablespoons blue cheese crumbles

Preheat grill pan to medium-high.

Cook steak about 6 minutes per side, seasoning each side with salt and pepper.

In a large bowl, mix tomatoes, onion, and garlic.

Let meat rest for 3 to 5 minutes after cooking, then slice across the grain and diagonally into thin strips.

Add meat and lettuce to bowl, pour on vinaigrette, and toss well so that everything is completely coated. Top with cheese.

Serves 2

Nutritional information, per serving: 293 calories, 33 g protein, 16 g carbs, 13 g total fat, 5 g saturated fat, 629 mg sodium, 4 g fiber

Searing to New Heights

Powerfoods: 2

2	(6-ounce) sirloin steaks	1	clove garlic, crushed
	Salt and pepper	¼	cup chicken broth
1	teaspoon olive oil	½	cup thinly sliced cremini mushrooms
¼	teaspoon dried thyme		

Sear steaks in a skillet heated over medium-high (about 2 to 3 minutes per side). Season each side with a pinch of salt and pepper as it cooks. Remove steaks from skillet. Reduce heat to medium.

Add oil, thyme, and garlic to skillet, stirring frequently and scraping with a spoon to release the brown bits left behind by the meat (about 30 seconds).

Add stock and mushrooms, stirring frequently until mushrooms soften (about 3 minutes). Serve over the steaks.

Serves 2

Nutritional information, per serving: 271 calories, 40 g protein, 2 g carbs, 11 g total fat, 4 g saturated fat, 141 mg sodium, 0 g fiber

My Mighty Mignon
Powerfoods: 5

1 zucchini, sliced	2 teaspoons olive oil
1 portobello mushroom cap, sliced	1 tablespoon balsamic vinegar
1 jar (5 ounces) artichoke halves, drained	2 (4 ounces each) filet mignons
2 green onions, cut into 1" pieces	Salt and pepper

Put vegetables, oil, and vinegar into a large zip-top plastic bag and shake well to coat. Set aside for 1 minute or 1 hour.

Sprinkle filets with salt and pepper, then place them on a medium-hot grill pan. Turn after 3 minutes, then cook for 3 minutes more for medium-rare.

Turn filets again, and slide them to side of pan. Add vegetables. Cook for 3 to 5 minutes more, stirring frequently.

Serves 2

Nutritional information, per serving: 262 calories, 29 g protein, 10 g carbs, 12 g total fat, 3 g saturated fat, 220 mg sodium, 3 g fiber

SEE RED

How can filet mignon fit into a diet? Easy. First, filet is cut from the tenderloin, one of the leanest cuts of beef. Second, notice the 4-ounce serving. That's 4 ounces of velvety soft, rich, flavorful beef—not 20 ounces of unsatisfying leathery porterhouse like you'd get from one of those joints in a shopping mall parking lot.

Salmon Says

Powerfoods: 2

1   tablespoon blueberry jam or jelly

2   teaspoons barbecue sauce

2   (4 ounces each) salmon fillets

Salt and pepper to taste

Preheat oven to broil.

In a small bowl, stir together jam and barbecue sauce until well blended.

Coat a baking sheet with cooking spray. Arrange salmon on it, sprinkle with salt and pepper, then spoon one-third of the sauce over each fillet. Reserve one-third.

Broil for 5 minutes or until fish flakes. Spoon remaining sauce over fillets before serving.

Serves 2

Nutritional information, per serving: 193 calories, 23 g protein, 8 g carbs, 7 g total fat, 1 g saturated fat, 78 mg sodium, 0 g fiber

Shrimp Boast

Powerfoods: 5

2 ounces Barilla Plus penne pasta

12–14 medium precooked, peeled shrimp

3 cups chopped baby spinach

1 tomato, chopped

3 tablespoons Gorgonzola cheese crumbles

2 tablespoons diced walnuts

3 tablespoons ready-made pesto

Cook pasta according to package directions. If you're using frozen shrimp, defrost them by running warm water over them.

Drain pasta.

Transfer pasta to a large bowl and add remaining ingredients, stirring well to help wilt the spinach and mix in the pesto.

Serves 2

Nutritional information, per serving: 372 calories, 19 g protein, 29 g carbs, 21 g total fat, 5 g saturated fat, 488 mg sodium, 5 g fiber

Tilapia Dance
Powerfoods: 5

1 tablespoon olive oil	2 (3–4 ounces each) tilapia fillets
½ teaspoon red pepper flakes	2 green onions, sliced
2 cups baby spinach, lightly packed	½ lime
10–12 asparagus tips	Salt and pepper

In a small bowl, mix oil and red pepper flakes. Microwave for 30 seconds to make chile oil. Set aside.

Tear off two 18" sections of foil and smooth flat. Arrange an equal amount of spinach and asparagus in the center of each piece of foil. Place fillets on top of each pile. Then top each fillet with equal amounts of green onion and chile oil.

Cut a half lime in half, and squeeze juice from each quarter over fish. Season with a pinch of salt and pepper, then seal (fold foil up and over fillets, then crease sides to form a tent).

Bake in a 450°F oven for 10 to 12 minutes.

Serves 2

Nutritional information, per serving: 218 calories, 22 g protein, 15 g carbs, 8 g total fat, 1 g saturated fat, 943 mg sodium, 6 g fiber

Marco Pollo
Powerfoods: 4

2 (4–5 ounces each) chicken breasts, pounded to an even ¼" thickness

Salt and pepper

1 teaspoon olive oil

1 clove garlic, crushed

½ teaspoon dried basil

¾ cup chopped zucchini

¾ cup canned no-salt-added tomatoes

Sear chicken in a skillet on medium-high heat (about 4 to 5 minutes per side). Season each side with a pinch of salt and pepper. Remove breasts from skillet. Reduce heat to medium.

Add oil and garlic to skillet, stirring frequently and scraping with a spoon to release the brown bits left behind by the chicken (about 30 seconds).

Add basil and zucchini. Let rest for 1 minute.

Stir in tomatoes, and return chicken breasts to skillet.

Cover and cook for 2 minutes. Optional: Top with Parmesan cheese just before serving.

Serves 2

Nutritional information, per serving: 174 calories, 28 g protein, 5 g carbs, 4 g total fat, 1 g saturated fat, 113 mg sodium, 1 g fiber

Chili-Chunked Chicken
Powerfoods: 3

1½ tablespoons Grillmates grill seasoning

8 chicken breast tenders

2½ cups red chili beans, drained and rinsed

1 cup canned no-salt-added diced tomatoes with chiles

¼ cup barbecue sauce

⅓ cup reduced-sodium chicken broth

¼ cup grated low-fat smoked Cheddar or Gouda cheese

Smear seasoning over chicken, then sear tenders in a medium-hot nonstick skillet coated with cooking spray. Cook for about 2 minutes per side.

Reduce heat to low; add beans, tomatoes, barbecue sauce, and broth. Stir well to blend.

Let the mixture simmer for 10 minutes, stirring occasionally. When ready to serve, top with cheese.

Serves 2

Nutritional information, per serving: 436 calories, 49 g protein, 56 g carbs, 2 g total fat, 1 g saturated fat, 1,471 mg sodium, 13 g fiber

ABS FACT

Convenience foods, like canned beans, come at a high sodium cost. (Something has to keep the beans from rotting on the shelf, and sodium does the trick.) Rinsing the beans well before you use them removes up to 40 percent of the sodium.

Guiltless Wings

Powerfoods: 2

3	tablespoons hot sauce	1	clove garlic, crushed
3	teaspoons honey	12	boneless, skinless chicken tenders
2	tablespoons low-sodium Worcestershire sauce		Low-fat blue cheese dressing
½	teaspoon paprika		

Preheat nonstick skillet to medium-high.

In a small bowl, stir together hot sauce, honey, Worcestershire sauce, paprika, and garlic until well blended. If the honey clumps, nuke the mixture for 10 to 15 seconds, then stir.

Place chicken and half the sauce mixture inside a large zip-top plastic bag, then shake to coat each piece.

Pour soaked tenders into the skillet and cook for 1 to 2 minutes per side. When done, toss with remaining sauce mixture to coat. Serve with dressing.

Serves 2

Nutritional information, per serving (without dressing): 217 calories, 41 g protein, 13 g carbs, 1 g total fat, 0 g saturated fat, 630 mg sodium, 0 g fiber

Penne for Your Thoughts

Powerfoods: 6

- 2 ounces Barilla Plus penne pasta
- 2 (4–5 ounces each) chicken breasts, pounded to ¼" thickness

  Salt and pepper to taste
- 1 teaspoon olive oil
- 1 clove garlic, crushed
- ½ teaspoon finely diced dried rosemary

- 1 cup cannellini beans, rinsed
- 2 heaping tablespoons diced roasted red pepper
- 4 cups baby spinach leaves
- 2 tablespoons grated Parmesan cheese

Cook pasta according to package directions.

While pasta is boiling, sear chicken in a skillet on medium-high heat (about 4 to 5 minutes per side), seasoning each side with a pinch of salt and pepper. Remove the breasts from the skillet and set aside.

Turn down heat to medium. Add oil, garlic, rosemary, beans, red pepper, and spinach to skillet. Cook until spinach wilts (about 1 to 2 minutes), turning frequently.

Slice chicken and toss it together with drained pasta and spinach-bean mixture. Top each plate with 1 tablespoon cheese.

Serves 2

Nutritional information, per serving: 412 calories, 42 g protein, 45 g carbs, 7 g total fat, 2 g saturated fat, 423 mg sodium, 9 g fiber

Six Degrees to Heaven Bacon

Powerfoods: 4

2 ounces Barilla Plus spaghetti

6 strips turkey bacon, chopped

1 egg

2 tablespoons grated Parmesan cheese

1 tablespoon olive oil

Cook pasta according to package directions.

While pasta is boiling, fry bacon in a nonstick skillet on medium-high heat (about 4 minutes). Remove from heat, and drain.

In a small bowl, whisk egg until well blended. Drain cooked pasta, then stir in egg (hot pasta will cook the egg), cheese, bacon, and oil. Toss well to mix.

Serves 2

Nutritional information, per serving: 323 calories, 16 g protein, 20 g carbs, 20 g total fat, 5 g saturated fat, 634 mg sodium, 2 g fiber

Under the Maple Treats

Powerfoods: 2

2 tablespoons maple syrup

2 tablespoons Dijon mustard

1 teaspoon olive oil

1 small clove garlic, crushed

Salt and pepper to taste

2 bone-in pork chops

Preheat cast-iron skillet to medium-high.

In a small bowl, stir together syrup, mustard, oil, garlic, salt, and pepper until well blended. Place chops and mustard mixture inside a large zip-top plastic bag, then shake to coat the chops.

Place chops on skillet, cooking 3 to 4 minutes per side. In last minute of cooking, pour remaining mustard mixture onto chops as they cook.

Serves 2

Nutritional information, per serving: 294 calories, 23 g protein, 17 g carbs, 16 g total fat, 5 g saturated fat, 403 mg sodium, 0 g fiber

Greek Balls of Fire

Powerfoods: 6

2	ounces Barilla Plus spaghetti	2	cloves garlic
5	ounces ground turkey breast	1	egg, whisked
2	tablespoons chopped fresh parsley	2	teaspoons olive oil
2	tablespoons feta cheese crumbles	2	cups marinara sauce

Cook pasta according to package directions.

While pasta is boiling, mix together turkey, parsley, feta, garlic, and egg in a large bowl until well blended. Roll into 1"-diameter meatballs.

Add oil to a nonstick skillet heated to medium-high heat. Cook meatballs for 4 minutes per side or until nicely browned.

Nuke marinara. Drain cooked pasta, and top with marinara and meatballs.

Serves 2

Nutritional information, per serving: 425 calories, 31 g protein, 41 g carbs, 16 g total fat, 4 g saturated fat, 1,225 mg sodium, 6 g fiber

Lemon Law

Powerfoods: 2

1 tablespoon + 2 teaspoons olive oil	¼ cup each: fresh parsley, mint, basil
1 large chicken breast	Salt and pepper to taste
½ lemon, juiced and zested	¼ cup white wine

Add 1 tablespoon oil to ovenproof skillet heated to medium-high heat. Place chicken in skillet, and sear for 2 minutes per side.

While chicken cooks, add remaining 2 teaspoons oil, lemon juice, zest, and herbs to blender or small food processor and pulse until well mixed.

Place skillet with chicken into a 400°F oven to roast for 8 minutes.

Remove skillet from oven, and place chicken on plate. Season to taste with salt and pepper.

Pour wine into hot skillet, scraping up any brown bits from bottom of pan. Pour in herb sauce and cook on stovetop for 1 minute more, stirring frequently. Pour sauce over chicken.

Serves 1

Nutritional information, per serving: 398 calories, 28 g protein, 6 g carbs, 24 g total fat, 4 g saturated fat, 93 mg sodium, 2 g fiber

Social Study: 60-Minute Special-Occasion Meals

There's nothing in the playbook that says just because it's a holiday or a family reunion or time for a candelit dinner that you have to hide your Abs Diet in the closet. Embrace it, show it off, cook for the crew. And make every meal a power meal.

Roast Beast

Powerfoods: 1

3 pounds sirloin roast	3 teaspoons salt
6 cloves garlic, crushed	1 tablespoon black pepper

Trim any remaining fat from beef, then rub with garlic. Sprinkle on salt and pepper, patting with your hands to help it stick to the beef.

Place roast on a broiler pan and bake at 450°F for 20 minutes. Reduce heat to 300° and cook for an additional 40 minutes (beef will be medium rare). Double-check internal temperature with a meat thermometer (should read 145°F).

Eat with baked potatoes and steamed green beans.

Serves 12

Nutritional information, per serving: 190 calories, 24 g protein, 1 g carbs, 10 g total fat, 4 g saturated fat, 641 mg sodium, 0 g fiber

Not-So-Big Bird

Powerfoods: 2

3–5 pounds turkey breast   Olive oil (for basting)

   Salt and pepper to taste

Rub turkey with salt and pepper.

Place turkey on a broiler pan and bake at 450°F for 45 minutes. Every 15 minutes, brush the bird with olive oil to keep it moist. Double-check internal temperature with a meat thermometer (should read 160°F).

Eat with cranberry sauce and green bean casserole.

Serves 6

Nutritional information, per serving: 168 calories, 37 g protein, 0 g carbs, 1 g total fat, 0 g saturated fat, 74 mg sodium, 0 g fiber

FREQUENTLY ABS QUESTION

ARE THERE ANY SUPPLEMENTS THAT CAN HELP WITH WEIGHT LOSS?

Conjugated linoleic acid (CLA) is a fatty acid that's been shown to aid in weight loss. Researchers reported that subjects taking CLA for 1 year lost up to 8.7 percent of their body fat. The recommended daily dose is 3 grams. And pyruvate is an antioxidant that may help aid weight loss. In two trials, taking pyruvate in addition to eating a low-fat diet stepped up weight loss. The recommended daily dosage is 25 grams.

Apple and Sausage Stuffing

Powerfoods: 5

1 pound turkey sausage	2 apples, chopped
8 cups cubed whole wheat bread, lightly toasted	2 tablespoons chopped fresh basil
2 teaspoons olive oil	1 teaspoon salt
4 cups chopped onions	1 teaspoon pepper
2 cups chopped celery	1½ cups low-fat, low-sodium chicken broth
2 cups chopped carrots	

Remove sausage from casings and brown in a nonstick skillet on medium-high heat (about 5 minutes). Remove from pan and add to bread cubes in a large bowl.

Using same pan, add oil and sauté onions, celery, and carrots until tender (about 10 minutes).

Add apples, basil, salt, and pepper, and sauté 5 minutes more.

Add vegetable-apple mixture to sausage and bread, tossing well to combine. Pour in broth, and stir well so bread soaks up the broth.

Coat a 13" x 9" casserole dish with cooking spray and spoon in dressing. Cover with foil, and bake at 425°F for 20 minutes. Uncover and bake 15 minutes more or until top is crispy.

Serves 8

Nutritional information, per serving: 244 calories, 16 g protein, 31 g carbs, 7 g total fat, 2 g saturated fat, 837 mg sodium, 5 g fiber

EXCUSE-PROOF YOUR DIET

YOUR EXCUSE	YOUR TACTIC
Your Marriage. Studies show that people gain weight in the first few years of marriage.	Establish healthful routines you can do together to combat the natural tendency to get a little lazy around the house—a walk after dinner, a game of HORSE in the driveway, a game of horseplay in the bedroom.
Your Kids. It's easy to swipe excess fries and eat bad when their main staples are grilled cheese and pizza.	Rationalize. Your kids burn off calories because they're moving faster than a paparazzi chase car. You? The junk foods will get stored under your chin. Some tactics: Limit junk-food night to one night for your kids. Volunteer to coach, not watch, your kids' games. That'll keep you up and moving rather than sitting and videotaping.
Your Stress. Under stress, it's a lot easier to reach for convenient foods than fresh ones.	Pack snacks like high-fiber energy bars or single-serving bags of almonds or other nuts to take the edge off during periods of high stress.
Your Happy Hour. Beer. Wings.	Eat a protein bar before going out, so you'll feel fuller. And drink a glass of water for every beer.

Good Going Gumbo

Powerfoods: 8

3 tablespoons olive oil

½ pound skinless, boneless chicken breasts, cut into bite-size pieces

1 pound low-fat turkey kielbasa, sliced into rounds

1½ cups chopped onion

1½ cups chopped green bell pepper

½ cup chopped celery

3 cloves garlic, crushed

½ teaspoon thyme

½ teaspoon paprika

½ teaspoon Creole seasoning

½ teaspoon pepper

⅓ cup flour

5 cups low-fat, low-sodium chicken broth

1 can (14.5 ounces) diced tomatoes

2 cups frozen sliced okra

1 pound fresh shrimp, peeled and deveined

Heat 1 tablespoon oil in a stock pot over medium heat. Add chicken and kielbasa and cook until browned (about 5 minutes). Remove chicken and kielbasa and set aside.

Add 1 tablespoon oil, onion, green pepper, celery, garlic, thyme, paprika, seasoning, and pepper to stock pot, and sauté until tender (about 10 minutes). Remove vegetables and add to chicken and kielbasa.

Add the remaining 1 tablespoon oil and the flour to stock pot, stirring with a whisk until flour is completely incorporated into oil.

Add broth, stirring well to blend.

Add chicken/vegetable mixture, along with tomatoes (with juice from can) and okra.

Bring to a boil, then reduce heat to low and simmer for 30 minutes.

Add shrimp and cook for 10 minutes until shrimp turns pink.

Eat with brown rice.

Serves 8

Nutritional information, per serving: 274 calories, 30 g protein, 18 g carbs, 9 g total fat, 2 g saturated fat, 718 mg sodium, 2 g fiber

Enchilada Lasagna

Powerfoods: 5

½ pound ground turkey breast

1½ cups reduced-fat Mexican-blend or Cheddar cheese

1 cup canned diced tomatoes, drained

1 cup low-fat, low-sodium cottage cheese

¼ cup canned jalapeño chile peppers, diced

½ cup green onions

2 teaspoons chili powder

2 cloves garlic, crushed

9 (6") corn tortillas

1 cup taco sauce

Brown turkey in a nonstick skillet (about 5 minutes).

Once cooled, combine with cheese (reserving ½ cup), tomatoes, cottage cheese, chiles, onions, chili powder, and garlic in a large bowl, stirring well to mix.

Coat an 11" x 7" baking dish with cooking spray. Place three tortillas on bottom of pan, and top with one-half of turkey mixture. Add three more tortillas, and top with remaining turkey mixture. Place three more tortillas on top, pour taco sauce over top tortillas, and sprinkle with remaining ½ cup cheese.

Bake at 375°F for 20 minutes.

Serves 4

Nutritional information, per serving: 437 calories, 34 g protein, 43 g carbs, 11 g total fat, 6 g saturated fat, 893 mg sodium, 3 g fiber

My Bolognese Has a First Name

Powerfoods: 7

- 2 tablespoons olive oil
- ¼ cup diced smoked turkey
- 1 carrot, peeled and diced
- 1 stalk celery, diced
- 1 small onion, diced
- 1 pound ground sirloin
- 2 cloves garlic, crushed
- ¾ cup red wine

- ¾ cup low-fat, no-sodium-added chicken broth
- 1 can (14 ounces) chopped tomatoes, drained
- ¼ cup low-fat milk
- 4 ounces Barilla Plus penne pasta
- 4 tablespoons grated reduced-fat mozzarella cheese

Heat oil in a large saucepan over medium heat. Add turkey, carrot, celery, and onion, and cook till very tender (about 10 minutes).

Add beef and garlic. Cook until beef is browned (about 5 minutes).

Add wine, stirring well, and cook for 10 minutes more.

Add broth, tomatoes, and milk, and simmer on medium-low heat for 30 minutes, stirring occasionally.

Prepare pasta according to package directions. Drain, then top with meat sauce and cheese.

Serves 4

Nutritional information, per serving: 485 calories, 35 g protein, 32 g carbs, 21 g total fat, 7 g saturated fat, 409 mg sodium, 4 g fiber

Meat Lover's Meat Loaf

Powerfoods: 4

½	pound ground sirloin	¾	cup diced onion
½	pound ground turkey breast	½	cup barbecue sauce, plus extra
2	eggs	2	cloves garlic, crushed
1	cup whole wheat crackers, crushed	½	teaspoon dried oregano

Mix the beef and turkey until well blended. Add eggs. Add remaining ingredients until well blended.

Form meat mixture into a loaf shape, and place onto a broiler pan. Coat with extra barbecue sauce.

Cook at 350°F for 1 hour. Double-check internal temperature with a meat thermometer (should read 160°F).

Eat with mashed potatoes.

Serves 4

Nutritional information, per serving: 366 calories, 32 g protein, 31 g carbs, 13 g total fat, 4 g saturated fat, 581 mg sodium, 3 g fiber

Apple-Cider Soaked Pork

Powerfoods: 1

1	pound pork tenderloin	2	cups apple cider
3	cloves garlic, crushed	½	cup balsamic or red wine vinegar

Place pork in an 11" x 7" baking dish, rub with garlic, and pour on cider and vinegar. Place in the refrigerator and marinate for 30 minutes.

Once grill is heated, grill tenderloin for 15 to 17 minutes. Double-check internal temperature with a meat thermometer (should read 160°F).

Eat with mashed spicy sweet potatoes. (Boil 4 small peeled sweet potatoes until tender, then mix with 1 teaspoon chili powder. Add fat-free half and half until you reach desired consistency.)

Serves 4

Nutritional information, per serving: 199 calories, 24 g protein, 16 g carbs, 4 g total fat, 1 g saturated fat, 70 mg sodium, 0 g fiber

Love Thee Tender

Powerfoods: 6

2   pounds pork tenderloin

1   cup reduced-fat ricotta cheese

½   teaspoon dried basil

2   cups chopped fresh baby spinach
    leaves

1   (5-ounce) jar artichoke hearts,
    drained and diced

Olive oil

Salt and pepper

Butterfly loin by splitting it down the center, cutting it almost but not completely through and then opening the two halves to lie flat and resemble a butterfly shape.

Stir cheese, basil, spinach, and artichokes together. Spread on the inside of cut loin. Roll the loin closed, and tie off with cord in at least five places.

Brush lightly with oil and sprinkle with salt and pepper.

Once grill is heated, grill tenderloin for 15 to 17 minutes. Double-check internal temperature with a meat thermometer (should read 160°F).

Eat with fire-roasted tomatoes (cut tomatoes in half and top with a sprinkle of basil, oregano, salt, and pepper). Arrange on a small baking sheet, place sheet on grill, shut grill lid, and cook for 5 to 10 minutes, until tomato peel looks slightly wilted.

Serves 8

Nutritional information, per serving: 183 calories, 28 g protein, 4 g carbs, 6 g total fat, 3 g saturated fat, 126 mg sodium, 1 g fiber

Bass in Net

Powerfoods: 2

1	lemon, juiced	1½	teaspoons cumin
2	cloves garlic, crushed	2	teaspoons pepper
½	teaspoon red pepper flakes	½	teaspoon salt
4	(6 ounces each) sea bass fillets	1	tablespoon olive oil
1½	teaspoons paprika		

In a zip-top plastic bag, mix together lemon juice, garlic, and red pepper flakes. Place fish in bag and refrigerate, marinating for 30 minutes.

In a small bowl, mix paprika, cumin, pepper, and salt, then rub mixture on each fillet.

Heat oil in a large nonstick skillet over medium heat. Add fillets, flesh-side down, and cook for 6 minutes. Flip and cook for 6 minutes more.

Eat with salad and lightly grilled bread.

Serves 4

Nutritional information, per serving: 210 calories, 32 g protein, 3 g carbs, 7 g total fat, 1 g saturated fat, 410 mg sodium, 1 g fiber

THE ABS DIET PROGRESS CHART

CATEGORY	WHAT IT MEANS	STARTING POINT	GOAL
Weight	While weighing yourself will help measure your progress, it's not the be-all number. That's because it doesn't take into account the amount of muscle you add—muscle weighs 20 percent more than fat, so even a dramatic fat loss may not translate into a dramatic weight loss at first.	_____	____
Body Mass Index (BMI)	It's a formula that takes into consideration your height and your weight and gives you an indication of whether you're overweight, obese, or in good shape. This measurement also doesn't include muscle mass or weight distribution, so it can be misleading. To figure it out, see below.	_____	____

BMI: To calculate BMI, multiply your weight in pounds by 703 and divide the number by your height in inches squared. A BMI of between 25 and 30 indicates you're overweight. Over 30 signifies obesity.

WAIST-TO-HIP RATIO: Measure your waist at your belly button and your hips at the widest point (around your butt). Divide your waist by your hips. You want a waist-to-hip ratio of 0.92 or lower.

CATEGORY	WHAT IT MEANS	STARTING POINT	GOAL
Waist-to-Hip Ratio	It approximates the amount of visceral fat you have—that's the kind of fat that pushes your waist out in front of you and threatens your organs. A lower waist-to-hip ratio means fewer health risks. See bottom of the opposite page for calculations.	_____	_____
Body-Fat Percentage	It takes into consideration your body composition—the percentage of body fat and muscle mass. Most methods require some bit of technology (a body-fat scale or calipers that measure body folds). See your gym for what options they may have. See below for an at-home version.	_____	_____

BODY-FAT PERCENTAGE: Sit in a chair with your feet flat on the floor. Gently pinch the skin on top of your thigh and measure the thickness of the pinched skin with a ruler. If it's ¾ inch or less, you probably have 14 percent body fat—ideal for a guy, quite fit for a woman. If it's 1 inch, you're probably closer to 18 percent, which is a little high for a man, but ideal for a woman. If you pinch more than an inch, you're at a higher risk for diseases associated with obesity, like diabetes and heart disease.

Chapter 8

PERFECT ABS
The Perfect Week of Eating

WE DID THE MATH so you don't have to. At least three servings of belly-blasting dairy daily? Yup. As many fruits and vegetables as you can cram down your craw? You bet. Whole grains galore? Got 'em—and more. This meal plan is designed to provide you with a steady stream of muscle-building protein and filling fiber throughout the day so you'll never get hungry.

The calorie calculations used to create the perfect week for men will help a sedentary guy in his mid-thirties lose 1 to 2 pounds. Each day's caloric total averages 2,000 calories. The perfect week for women, with 1,200 to 1,400 calories per day, will help his female counterpart lose up to 2 pounds.

Not sedentary? Good—you should have no problem hitting this weight-loss goal.

Perfect Week for Men

MONDAY

Breakfast

Guac Your World (page 88)

8 ounces orange juice

Smoothie

Dark Vader (page 151)

Lunch

Welcome to Monterey, Jack (page 101)

1 ounce reduced-fat or baked potato chips

Water or unsweetened tea

Snack

¾ cup broccoli or carrots

2 tablespoons Spread Yourself Thin (page 163)

Dinner

Chicken Little Italy (page 130)

1 whole wheat roll

8 ounces fruit juice

Dessert

Yogi Pops (page 171)

TUESDAY

Breakfast

Breakfast with Barbie (page 82)

8 ounces fat-free milk

Smoothie

Belly-Busting Berry (page 148)

Lunch

Mesquite Bites (page 108)

1 whole wheat roll

Water or unsweetened tea

Snack

Berry Up to the Bar (page 164)

Dinner

Heavenly Honolulu (page 144)

12 ounces light beer

Dessert

Low-fat ice cream sandwich

WEDNESDAY

Breakfast

The Swiss-Army Sandwich (page 89)

8 ounces orange juice

Smoothie

Show Me the Honey (page 152)

Lunch

Reuben Reduced (page 100)

1 cup mixed fruit

8 ounces fat-free milk

Snack

1 ounce almonds

Dinner

Jump for Soy (page 134)

See Slaw (page 157)

Dessert

1 carton low-fat yogurt with fruit

THURSDAY

Breakfast

A Breakfast to Relish (page 93)

8 ounces fat-free milk

Smoothie

Blue Cheesecake (page 151)

Lunch

The Melon Banquet (page 107)

1 whole wheat roll

Water or unsweetened tea

Snack

PB Power Apples (page 165)

Dinner

Chop Chop! (page 119)

Water or unsweetened tea

Dessert

Low-fat pudding cup

FRIDAY

Breakfast

The Lite Lumberjack (page 81)

8 ounces fruit juice

Smoothie

Extreme Chocolate (page 150)

Lunch

Egg Yourself On (page 101)

1 ounce reduced-fat or baked potato chips

Water or unsweetened tea

Snack

2 slices lunchmeat

1 slice reduced-fat cheese

Dinner

Slammin' Salmon (page 126)

Water or unsweetened tea

Dessert

Berried Alive (page 169)

SATURDAY

Breakfast

Raisin the Stakes (page 85)

8 ounces orange juice

Smoothie

Strawberry Shortcut (page 149)

Lunch

Crunch Time (page 105)

Water or unsweetened tea

Snack

1 carton low-fat yogurt with fruit

Dinner

Spinach City (page 142)

12 ounces light beer

Dessert

Your Sundae Best (page 172)

SUNDAY

Breakfast

Mint Condition (page 80)

8 ounces orange juice

Smoothie

Coco Poof (page 149)

Lunch

Join the Club (page 100)

8 ounces fruit juice

Snack

1 ounce almonds

1 stick string cheese

Dinner

Cheat Meal

Perfect Week for Women

MONDAY

Breakfast

Change Your Tuna (page 93)

Unsweetened tea or coffee

Smoothie

½ Belly-Busting Berry (page 148)

Lunch

Crunch Time (page 105)

Water or unsweetened tea

Snack

Cucumber Tubes (page 168)

Dinner

Gone Fishing (page 125)

Water or unsweetened tea

Dessert

Low-fat ice cream sandwich

TUESDAY

Breakfast

Mint Condition (page 80)

Unsweetened tea or coffee

Smoothie

½ Show Me the Honey (page 152)

Lunch

Roll of a Lifetime (page 103)

Water or unsweetened tea

Snack

1 stick string cheese

5–7 whole wheat crackers, such as Triscuits

Dinner

Terra Ricotta (page 140)

Water or unsweetened tea

Dessert

Yogi Pops (page 171)

WEDNESDAY

Breakfast

Mo' Feta, Mo' Betta (page 95)

Unsweetened tea or coffee

Smoothie

½ Extreme Chocolate (page 150)

Lunch

Popeye and Olive Oil (page 109)

Water or unsweetened tea

Snack

½ PB Power Apples (page 165)

Dinner

Colonel Mustard (page 129)

Water or unsweetened tea

Dessert

Low-fat ice cream sandwich

THURSDAY

Breakfast
Waffles Rancheros (page 89)

Smoothie
½ Pumpkin You Up! (page 150)

Lunch
Reuben Reduced (page 100)

Water or unsweetened tea

Snack
1 stick string cheese

5–7 whole wheat crackers, such as Triscuits

Dinner
The Orange and Gold (page 116)

Water or unsweetened tea

Dessert
Yogi Pops (page 171)

FRIDAY

Breakfast

Breakfast with Barbie (page 82)

Smoothie

½ Coco Poof (page 149)

Lunch

The Melon Banquet (page 107)

Water or unsweetened tea

Snack

Cucumber Tubes (page 168)

Dinner

Chicken Little Italy (page 130)

Water or unsweetened tea

Dessert

1 carton low-fat yogurt with fruit

SATURDAY

Breakfast

Corn to Be Wild (page 94)

Smoothie

½ Belly-Busting Berry (page 148)

Lunch

The Two Chicks (page 106)

Water or unsweetened tea

Snack

2 tablespoons Spread Yourself Thin (page 163)

¾ cup broccoli or carrots

Dinner

Shrimp to Nuts (page 123)

Water or unsweetened tea

Dessert

Yogi Pops (page 171)

SUNDAY

Breakfast

The 'Bama Bowl (page 82)

Smoothie

½ Lemon Drips and Drops (page 152)

Lunch

Pimp My Shrimp (page 107)

Water or unsweetened tea

Snack

½ Lemon Drips and Drops (page 152)

Dinner

Cheat meal

The Abs Diet Bull's-Eye

Variety being the spice of life and all, you're often going to have the opportunity and the desire to mix in foods that don't fall squarely into the ABS DIET POWER 12. That's fine, as long as you keep your eye on the target and try to mix at least two Powerfoods into each meal and snack.

To help keep you focused on the ABS DIET POWER 12, I've created a little game I call the Abs Diet Bull's-Eye. In the center of this chart are the foods you want to concentrate on. Around them, in concentric layers, are additional foods you'll no doubt run across every day.

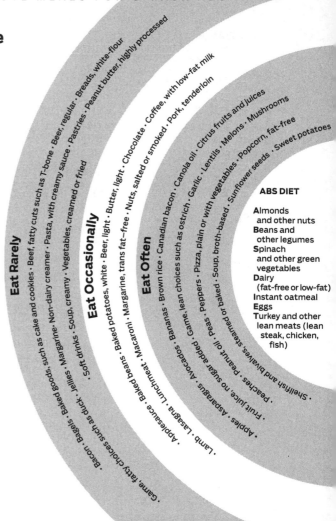

Eat Rarely

Bacon · Bagels · Baked goods, such as cake and cookies · Beef, fatty cuts such as T-bone · Beer, regular · Breads, white-flour · Pastries · Peanut butter, highly processed

Eat Occasionally

Game, fatty choices such each duck · Soft drinks · Jellies · Margarine · Non-dairy creamer · Pasta, with creamy sauce · Vegetables, creamed or fried

Eat Often

Applesauce · Baked beans · Baked potatoes, white · Beer, light · Butter, light · Chocolate · Coffee, with low-fat milk · Nuts, salted or smoked · Pork, tenderloin

Apples · Asparagus · Avocados · Bananas · Brown rice · Canadian bacon · Canola oil · Citrus fruits and juices · Lamb · Lasagna · Luncheat · Macaroni · Margarine, trans fat–free · Game, lean choices such as ostrich · Garlic · Lentils · Melons · Mushrooms · Peaches · peanut oil · Peas · Peppers · Pizza, plain or with vegetables · Popcorn, fat-free · Fruit juice no sugar added · Shellfish and bivalves, steamed or baked · Soup, broth-based · Sunflower seeds · Sweet potatoes

ABS DIET

Almonds
and other nuts
Beans and
other legumes
Spinach
and other green
vegetables
Dairy
(fat-free or low-fat)
Instant oatmeal
Eggs
Turkey and other
lean meats (lean
steak, chicken,
fish)

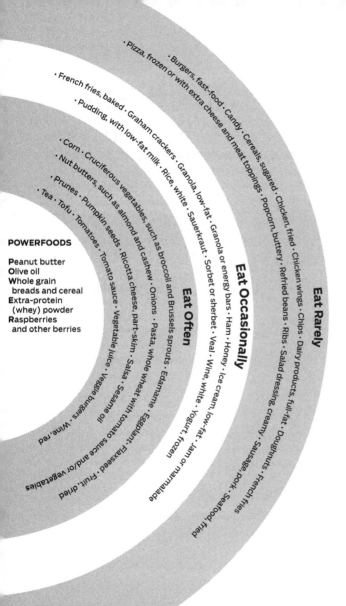

POWERFOODS

Peanut butter
Olive oil
Whole grain
breads and cereal
Extra-protein
(whey) powder
Raspberries
and other berries

Eat Often

Eat Occasionally

Eat Rarely

· Corn · Cruciferous vegetables, such as broccoli and Brussels sprouts · Edamame · Eggplant · Flaxseed · Fruit, dried · Vegetable juice · Veggie burgers · Wine, red

· Nut butters, such as almond and cashew · Onions · Pasta, whole wheat with tomato sauce and/or vegetables

· Prunes · Pumpkin seeds · Ricotta cheese, part-skim · Salsa · Sesame oil

· Tea · Tofu · Tomatoes · Tomato sauce · Vegetable juice · Veggie burgers · Wine, red

· Pudding, with low-fat milk · Rice, white · Sauerkraut · Sorbet or sherbet · Veal · Wine, white · Yogurt, frozen

· French fries, baked · Graham crackers · Granola, low-fat · Granola or energy bars · Ham · Honey · Ice cream, low-fat · Jam or marmalade

· Pizza, frozen or with extra cheese and meat toppings · Popcorn, buttery · Refried beans · Ribs · Salad dressing, creamy · Sausage · Seafood, fried

· Burgers, fast-food · Candy · Cereals, sugared · Chicken, fried · Chicken wings · Chips · Dairy products, full-fat · Doughnuts · French fries

Indulge in them from time to time, but try to stay as focused on the center of the bull's-eye as you can. You have the flexibility to eat what you want, but this bull's-eye will help you focus on the center goal. The closer you stick to the inside, the healthier your diet will be and the better results you'll see. And if your dinnertime darts are always hitting outside the ring, then I think you may need to reevaluate your form.

THE ABS DIET EXERCISE CHEAT SHEET

SUBJECT	GUIDELINE
Number of workouts	3 per week
Strength training	Circuits emphasizing your biggest muscle groups, like your legs, back, and chest. Total-body circuits can be done in 20 minutes three times a week for muscle-building and fat-burning. See the opposite page for the original Abs Diet Circuit.
Cardiovascular training	One high-intensity interval workout a week (after one of your strength workouts). Perform cardiovascular exercise with periods of high intensity and periods of low intensity or rest. The change helps boost your metabolism and burn more calories.
Abdominal exercises	Do a circuit of 5 or 6 exercises, emphasizing different parts of your abdominal region (including your lower back). Do it at the beginning of two of your strength workouts. See page 238 for sample exercises.
Equipment needed	Dumbbells. Optional: bench, stability ball
Advanced programs	See the book *The Abs Diet Get Fit, Stay Fit Plan* for hundreds of exercises and dozens of plans.

THE ABS DIET ORIGINAL CIRCUIT: THE AT-HOME VERSION

DO THE EXERCISES on the next four pages in the following manner: Perform one set of an exercise and then move immediately to the next exercise, with no more than 30 seconds of rest. When you complete one circuit—that is, a set of every exercise—rest for 2 minutes, then complete a second circuit of the non-abs exercises.

EXERCISE	HOW TO DO IT	REPS	SETS
5–6 abs exercises	See page 238 or the book *The Abs Diet Get Fit, Stay Fit Plan* for ideas.	15–20 of each	1
Squat	Stand with one dumbbell in each hand. Set your feet shoulder-width apart; keep your knees slightly bent, back straight, and eyes focused straight ahead. Slowly lower your body as if you were sitting back into a chair, keeping your back naturally aligned and your lower legs nearly perpendicular to the floor. When your thighs are parallel to the floor, pause, then return to the starting position.	10–12	2
Pushup	Get in a pushup position with your hands shoulder-width apart. Bend at the elbows while keeping your back straight until your chin almost touches the floor, then push back up. Do them on your knees if standard ones are too difficult.	10–12	2
Bent-over row	Stand with your knees slightly bent and shoulder-width apart. Bend forward so that your back is almost parallel to the floor. Holding a dumbbell in each hand, let your arms hang toward the floor. With your palms facing in, pull the dumbbells toward you until they touch the outside of your chest. Pause, then return to the starting position.	10	2

EXERCISE	HOW TO DO IT	REPS	SETS
Military press	Sitting in a sturdy chair or on a bench, hold one dumbbell in each hand, about level with your ears. Push the dumbbells straight overhead so that your arms are almost fully extended, hold for a count of one, then return to the starting position.	10	2
Upright row	Grab a dumbbell with each hand and stand with your feet shoulder-width apart and your knees slightly bent. Let the weights hang at arm's length on top of your thighs. Bending your elbows, lift your upper arms straight out to the sides; pull the dumbbells straight up until your upper arms are parallel to the floor and the weights are just below chin level. Pause, then return to the starting position.	10	2
Triceps kickback	Grab a dumbbell with each hand and stand with your knees slightly bent and shoulder-width apart. Bend over so that your back is almost parallel to the ground. Bend your elbows to about 90-degree angles, raising them to just above the level of your back. This is the starting position. Extend your forearms backward, keeping your upper arms stationary. When they're fully extended, your arms should be parallel to the ground. Pause, then return to the starting position.	10–12	2

(continued)

EXERCISE	HOW TO DO IT	REPS	SETS
Wall squat	Stand with your back flat against a wall. Squat down so your thighs are parallel to the ground (higher if you can't go that far). Hold that position for as long as you can. That's one set. Aim for 20 seconds to start, and work your way up to 45 seconds.	10–12	2
Biceps curl	Stand, holding a dumbbell in each hand, palms facing out, with your hands shoulder-width apart and your arms hanging in front of you. Curl the weight toward your shoulders, hold for 1 second, then return to the starting position.	10	2
Leg curl	Lie down with your stomach on the floor. Put a light dumbbell between your feet (so that the top end of the dumbbell rests on the bottom of your feet). Squeeze your feet together, and curl them toward your butt.	10–12	2

EXERCISE	HOW TO DO IT	REPS	SETS
Traveling lunge	Holding a dumbbell in each hand with your arms at your sides, stand with your feet hip-width apart at one end of the room; you need space to walk about 20 steps. (If your available exercise area is not big enough for this, you can do the exercise in one place, alternating your lead foot wth each lunge.) Step forward with your left foot, and lower your body so that your left thigh is parallel to the floor and your right thigh is perpendicular to the floor. (Your right knee should bend and almost touch the floor.) Stand and bring your right foot up next to your left, then repeat with the right leg lunging forward.	10–12 each leg	2
Step-up	Stand facing a staircase and place your left foot on the bottom step so that your knee is bent at 90 degrees. Your knee should not advance past the toes of your left foot. Push off with your left foot, and bring your right foot onto the step, keeping your back straight. Now step down with the left foot, followed by the right. Alternate the leading foot, or do all of the repetitions leading with one foot and then alternating. Once you're comfortable, add dumbbells.	10–12 each leg	2

A 6-PACK OF EXERCISES FOR A 6-PACK OF ABS

Beginner

SUPERMAN

Lie facedown on the floor with your legs straight and your arms extended straight forward (as though you were signaling a touchdown and fell on your face). Simultaneously lift your shoulders, legs, and arms off the floor. Hold as long as you can, working up to 60 seconds.

NEGATIVE CRUNCH

Sit with your knees bent and your feet flat on the floor, shoulder-width apart. (Tuck your feet under weights to maintain balance.) Extend your arms in front of you with your fingers interlaced. Begin with your upper body at slightly less than a 90-degree angle to the floor. Now round your lower back and, with your abs contracted, lower your torso toward the floor. When your upper body reaches a 45-degree angle to the floor, return to the starting position. Do 10 to 15 repetitions.

Intermediate

SWISS BALL PLANK

Assume a modified pushup position with your feet on the floor and your elbows resting on a Swiss ball. Once you feel balanced, raise one foot a few inches off the floor and hold for 6 seconds. Place the foot back on the floor and lift the other for 6 seconds. That's 1 repetition. Do 6.

MED BALL KNEE RAISE

Lie faceup on the floor with your hands behind your ears, your feet on the floor, and a medicine ball held between bent knees. Keeping your lower back on the floor, contract your abdominals and pull your knees toward your chest. Lower your knees to the left, bring them back to the center, then return to the starting position. On the next repetition, drop your knees to the right, and alternate sides for each rep. Do three sets of 12 repetitions.

Advanced

ALTERNATING PLANK

Widen your hands and feet from the standard pushup position, then walk your hands out a couple of inches ahead of your shoulders. Lift your left leg and right arm and hold for 10 seconds. Lower and repeat, switching sides. That's 1 repetition. Do 6.

SCISSOR-KICK CRUNCH

Lie faceup on the floor with your legs straight. Lift your legs 30 degrees off the floor and spread them. Crunch forward. As you crunch up and forward, move your left leg under and past your right leg, then back. Repeat, switching legs. The cadence will come to you with practice, so don't count repetitions; just repeat for 30 seconds.

NUTRITIONAL VALUES OF COMMON FOODS

THE NEW TREND TOWARD LOW-CARB DIETS has a lot of us eating plenty of fat and protein. But many of us are missing out on the valuable micronutrients found in whole grains, fruits, vegetables, and other foods that are verboten on a low-carb diet.

It might seem easier to ensure your daily value of nutrients by popping a multivitamin instead of eating a balanced diet. But there are two problems with nutrition that comes in a plastic container: First, multivitamins have no fiber, so this critical nutrient is missing if all you do is pop a pill for protection. Second, foods are loaded with plenty of nutrients beyond the standard vitamins C and E—and the importance of many of these nutrients, called phytochemicals, is only now being understood. "In a balanced diet, there are thousands of antioxidants. In pill form, you're just getting a few out of the thousands," says Edgar Miller, MD, PhD, of Johns Hopkins University in Baltimore.

To see how nutritionally complete your diet is, refer to the following chart for each food's vitamin and mineral values, and tally your total intake. If you come up short of the Recommended Dietary Allowances (RDAs), don't worry. Just eat more foods high in whatever vitamins or minerals you're lacking, and take a multivitamin/mineral supplement each day.

	VITAMIN A (MCG)	VITAMIN B₁ (THIAMIN) (MG)	VITAMIN B₆ (MG)	FOLATE (MCG)
RDAS FOR MEN/WOMEN	900/700	1.2/1.1	1.3/1.3	400/400
Almonds (1 oz)	0	0.05	0.03	11
Apple (1 medium)	8	0.02	0.06	4
Apricot (1)	67	0.01	0.02	3
Artichoke (1 medium)	0	0.10	0.15	87
Asparagus (1 medium spear)	12	0.02	0.01	8
Avocado (1)	122	0.20	0.60	124
Bacon (3 slices)	0	0.08	0.07	0.40
Bagel (4")	0	0.15	0.05	20
Banana (1 medium)	7	0.04	0.40	24
Beans, baked (1 cup)	13	0.40	0.34	61
Beans, black (1 cup cooked)	1	0.40	0.12	256
Beans, kidney (1 cup cooked)	0	0.28	0.21	230
Beans, lima (½ cup cooked)	32	0.12	0.16	22
Beans, navy (1 cup cooked)	0.36	0.40	0.30	255
Beans, pinto (1 cup cooked)	0	0.17	0.16	294
Beans, refried (1 cup)	0	0.07	0.36	28
Beans, white (1 cup cooked)	0	0.20	0.17	145

VITAMIN C (MG)	VITAMIN E (MG)	CALCIUM (MG)	MAGNESIUM (MG)	POTASSIUM (MG)	SELENIUM (MCG)	ZINC (MG)	CALORIES
90/75	15/15	1,000/1,000	420/320	4,700/4,700	55/55	11/8	
0	6	71	86	180	0	1	170
6	0.25	8	7	148	0	0.06	80
3.50	0.30	5	3.50	90	0.03	0.07	20
15	0.24	56	77	474	0.26	0.60	25
1	0.18	4	2	32	0.37	0.10	5
16	3	22	78	1,204	0.80	0.84	250
0	0.06	2	6	107	12	0.70	110
0	0.04	16	26	90	28	1	247
10	0.12	6	32	422	1	0.20	110
8	1.35	127	81	752	12	4	239
0	0.14	46	120	610	2	1.90	240
2	0.05	62	74	717	2	1.80	260
9	0.12	27	63	485	1.70	0.70	229
1.64	0.73	127	107	670	11	1.90	255
1.37	1.61	72	70	495	19	1.70	245
15	0	88	83	675	3	3	240
0	1.74	161	113	1,004	2.30	2.50	249

(continued)

	VITAMIN A (MCG)	VITAMIN B₁ (THIAMIN) (MG)	VITAMIN B₆ (MG)	FOLATE (MCG)
RDAS FOR MEN/WOMEN	900/700	1.2/1.1	1.3/1.3	400/400
Beef, ground lean (3 oz)	0	0.06	0.24	7
Beer (12 oz)	0	0.02	0.18	21
Beets (½ cup)	3	0.02	0.05	74
Blueberries (1 pint)	17	0.11	0.15	17
Bran, wheat (1 cup)	0	0.14	0.35	14
Bread, rye (1 slice)	0.26	0.14	0.02	35
Bread, white (1 slice)	0	0.11	0.02	28
Bread, whole grain (1 slice)	0	0.11	0.10	30
Breakfast sandwich, fast-food (bacon, egg, and cheese)	0	0.53	0.16	73
Broccoli (1 cup)	213	0.05	0.11	50
Brussels sprouts (½ cup)	60	0.08	0.14	47
Cake, coffee (1 piece)	20	0.10	0.03	27
Cake, frosted (1 piece)	10	0.01	0.02	7
Canadian bacon (2 slices)	0	0.40	0.20	2
Candy, non-chocolate (1 package)	0	0	0	0

VITAMIN C (MG)	VITAMIN E (MG)	CALCIUM (MG)	MAGNESIUM (MG)	POTASSIUM (MG)	SELENIUM (MCG)	ZINC (MG)	CALORIES
90/75	15/15	1,000/1,000	420/320	4,700/4,700	55/55	11/8	
0	0.15	7	19	265	0	4	185
0	0	18	21	89	2.50	0.04	153
3	0.03	11	16	221	0.50	0.24	29
28	1.65	17	17	223	0.30	0.50	165
0	0.54	26	220	426	28	3	120
0.13	0.11	23	13	53	10	0.36	83
0	0.06	38	6	25	4.30	0.20	67
0.08	0.09	24	14	53	8	0.30	65
2	0.60	160	25	211	36.0	2	441
66	0.33	34	18	230	2	0.30	20
48	0.34	28	16	247	1.17	0.26	28
0.11	0.11	76	10	63	9	0.25	180
0.04	0	18	14	84	1.40	0.30	239
0	0.16	5	10	181	11	0.80	137
0	0	0	0	0	0	0	230

(continued)

	VITAMIN A (MCG)	VITAMIN B₁ (THIAMIN) (MG)	VITAMIN B₆ (MG)	FOLATE (MCG)
RDAS FOR MEN/WOMEN	**900/700**	**1.2/1.1**	**1.3/1.3**	**400/400**
Cantaloupe (1 medium wedge)	345	0.04	0.07	21
Carrot (1)	734	0.04	0.08	12
Cauliflower (1 cup)	2	0.06	0.22	57
Celery (1 cup, strips)	55	0.03	0.10	45
Cereal, whole grain, with raisins (½ cup)	3	0.16	0.10	22
Cheddar cheese (1 slice)	75	0.01	0.02	5
Chef's salad with no dressing (1½ cups)	146	0.40	0.40	101
Cherries, sweet, raw (1 cup)	30	0.07	0.05	5.80
Chicken, skinless (½ breast)	4	0.04	0.32	2
Chickpeas (1 cup cooked)	4	0.19	0.22	282
Chili with beans (1 cup)	87	0.12	0.30	59
Chips, potato, lite (1 oz)	0	0.05	0.22	8
Chocolate (1.45 oz)	20	0.05	0.01	5
Cinnamon bun (1)	0	0.12	0	17
Citrus fruits and frozen concentrate juices (12 oz)	7	0.17	0.30	31

VITAMIN C (MG)	VITAMIN E (MG)	CALCIUM (MG)	MAGNESIUM (MG)	POTASSIUM (MG)	SELENIUM (MCG)	ZINC (MG)	CALORIES
90/75	15/15	1,000/1,000	420/320	4,700/4,700	55/55	11/8	
37	0.05	9	12	272	0.40	0.18	24
4	0.40	20	7	195	0.06	0.15	35
46	0.08	22	15	303	0.60	0.30	25
4	0.33	50	14	322	0.50	0.16	17
0.55	0.40	33	70	207	10	1	195
0	0.08	204	8	28	4	0.90	114
16	0	235	49	401	37	3	267
10	0.20	21	16	325	0.90	0.09	90
0.71	0.08	6.50	16	150	11	0.50	130
2	0.60	80	79	477	6	2.50	269
4	1.46	120	115	934	3	5	220
3.40	0.62	10	18	285	2	0.17	142
0	0.83	78	26	153	2	0.83	230
0.06	0.48	10	3.60	19	5	0.10	418
324	0.24	85	68	1,336	1	0.41	186

(continued)

	VITAMIN A (MCG)	VITAMIN B₁ (THIAMIN) (MG)	VITAMIN B₆ (MG)	FOLATE (MCG)
RDAS FOR MEN/WOMEN	900/700	1.2/1.1	1.3/1.3	400/400
Clams, fried (¾ cup)	101	0.11	0.07	41
Coffee (1 cup)	0	0	0	5
Collards (1 cup cooked)	1,542	0.08	0.24	177
Cookie, chocolate chip (1)	0.04	0.01	0.01	0.90
Corn (1 cup)	0.26	0.06	0.16	115
Cottage cheese, low-fat (1 cup)	25	0.05	0.15	27
Crackers (12)	0	0.17	0	0
Cranberry juice cocktail (1 cup)	1	0.02	0.05	0
Cream cheese (1 Tbsp)	53	0	0	2
Cucumber with peel (½ cup)	10	0.01	0.02	7
Doughnut (1)	17	0.10	0.03	24
Egg, whole (1 large)	84	0.03	0.06	22
Eggplant (1 cup)	4	0.08	0.09	14
English muffin, whole wheat (1)	0.09	0.25	0.05	36
Fig bar cookies (2 bars)	3	0.05	0.02	11
Fish, white (1 fillet)	60	0.26	0.50	26
French fries (10)	0	0.07	0.16	8

VITAMIN C (MG)	VITAMIN E (MG)	CALCIUM (MG)	MAGNESIUM (MG)	POTASSIUM (MG)	SELENIUM (MCG)	ZINC (MG)	CALORIES
90/75	15/15	1,000/1,000	420/320	4,700/4,700	55/55	11/8	
11.25	0	71	16	366	33	1.60	560
0	0.05	2	5	114	0	0.02	2
35	1.67	266	38	220	1	0.50	61
0	0.26	2.50	3	14	0	0.06	63
12	0.15	8	44	343	1.54	1.36	120
0	0.02	138	11	194	20	0.86	180
0	0	28	12	48	2.40	0.20	155
90	0	8	5	46	0	0.18	137
0	0.04	12	1	17	0.40	0.10	51
2.76	0	7	6	75	0	0.10	8
0.09	0.90	21	9	60	4	0.30	230
0	0.50	25	5	63	15	0.50	74
1	0.40	6	11	122	0.10	0.12	35
0	0.26	101	21	106	17	0.61	134
0.10	0.21	20	9	66	1	0.12	111
0	0.39	51	65	625	25	2	168
6	0.12	4	11	211	0.20	0.20	100

(continued)

	VITAMIN A (MCG)	VITAMIN B₁ (THIAMIN) (MG)	VITAMIN B₆ (MG)	FOLATE (MCG)
RDAS FOR MEN/WOMEN	**900/700**	**1.2/1.1**	**1.3/1.3**	**400/400**
Fruit, dried (1 oz)	208	0.01	0.05	1.1
Fruit juice, unsweetened (1 cup)	0	0.02	0.06	35
Garlic (1 clove)	0	0	0.04	0.09
Graham cracker (1 large rectangular piece)	0	0.03	0.01	6
Granola bar (1)	2	0.06	0.02	6
Grape juice (1 cup)	1	0.07	0.16	8
Ham (1 slice)	0	0.20	0.10	1
Hamburger, fast-food, with condiments and vegetables (1)	4	0.30	0.12	52
Hot dog, fast-food (1)	0	0.44	0.09	85
Ice cream (1 serving)	6	0.03	0.04	11
Jam or preserves (1 Tbsp)	0.20	0	0	2
Kale (1 cup)	955	0.07	0.11	18
Ketchup (1 Tbsp)	7	0	0.02	2
Kiwifruit (1 medium)	3	0.02	0.07	19
Lasagna, meat (7 oz)	61	0.19	0.20	16

VITAMIN C (MG)	VITAMIN E (MG)	CALCIUM (MG)	MAGNESIUM (MG)	POTASSIUM (MG)	SELENIUM (MCG)	ZINC (MG)	CALORIES
90/75	15/15	1,000/1,000	420/320	4,700/4,700	55/55	11/8	
1	0.31	11.82	11.13	226	0	0.14	69
40	0	160	9	154	0	0.20	117
0.90	0	5	0.75	12	0.40	0	4
0	0.05	3	4	19	1	0.10	59
0.22	0.32	15	24	82	4	0.50	117
0.25	0	23	25	334	0.25	0.13	154
0	0.10	2	5	94	6	0.50	30
2	0.42	126	23	251	20	2	512
0.09	0.10	108	27	190	29	2	242
0.46	0	72	19	164	1.65	0.40	133
2	0	4	0.80	15	0.40	0	56
33	1	180	23	417	1.17	0.23	39
2	0.20	3	3	57	0.04	0	15
70	1	26	13	237	0.15	0.10	50
12	0.94	220	41	372	28	3	318

(continued)

	VITAMIN A (MCG)	VITAMIN B$_1$ (THIAMIN) (MG)	VITAMIN B$_6$ (MG)	FOLATE (MCG)
RDAS FOR MEN/WOMEN	**900/700**	**1.2/1.1**	**1.3/1.3**	**400/400**
Lentils (1 cup cooked)	4.75	0.33	0.35	358
Lettuce, iceberg (1 cup)	8	0.02	0.03	31
Lettuce, romaine (½ cup)	81	0.02	0.02	38
Liver, beef (3 oz)	8,042	0.16	0.86	215
Lunchmeat, salami (3 slices)	0	0.10	0.08	0.34
Macaroni and cheese (8 oz)	48	0.25	0	0
Meat loaf (1 slice)	20	0.10	0.14	12
Melon, honeydew (1 cup)	5	0.07	0.16	34
Milk, fat-free (1 cup)	5	0.10	0.10	12
Milk, soy (1 cup)	0	0.15	0.16	40
Muffin, blueberry (1)	13	0.10	0.01	42
Mushrooms (1 cup sliced)	0	0.09	0.10	12
Nachos with cheese (6–8)	170	0.20	0.20	12
Nectarine (1)	23	0.05	0.03	7
Oatmeal (1 cup)	0.12	0.12	0.10	13
Olives (1 Tbsp)	1.70	0	0	0
Onion rings (10 medium)	0.98	0.10	0.07	64

VITAMIN C (MG)	VITAMIN E (MG)	CALCIUM (MG)	MAGNESIUM (MG)	POTASSIUM (MG)	SELENIUM (MCG)	ZINC (MG)	CALORIES
90/75	15/15	1,000/1,000	420/320	4,700/4,700	55/55	11/8	
0.22	2.97	37	71	731	5.54	2.51	230
2	0.02	11	4	84	0.28	0.10	8
7	0.04	9	4	69	0.10	0.06	5
1.62	0.43	5	18	300	31	4.50	162
0	0.05	1.34	2.86	63	4	0.54	150
0	0	102	0	111	0	0	415
0.62	0.10	43	22	295	0	4	231
32	0.04	11	18	403	1.24	0.16	61
2	0.10	301	27	406	5	1	83
0	0	80	60	440	3	0.90	100
0.63	0.47	32	9	70	6	0.30	158
2	0.10	5	10	355	8	0.70	15
1	0	311	63	196	18	2	296
7	1	8	12	273	0	0.23	70
0	0.26	19	51	175	0	1.43	150
0	0.14	7	0.30	0.67	0.08	0	10
0.68	0.39	86	19	152	3	0.41	370

(continued)

	VITAMIN A (MCG)	VITAMIN B$_1$ (THIAMIN) (MG)	VITAMIN B$_6$ (MG)	FOLATE (MCG)
RDAS FOR MEN/WOMEN	900/700	1.2/1.1	1.3/1.3	400/400
Oyster (1 medium)	4.20	0.01	0.01	1.40
Pancakes (2)	7.60	0.16	0.07	28
Pasta with red sauce (4.5 oz)	0	0.13	0.10	4
Peach (1 medium)	16	0.02	0.02	4
Peanut butter (2 Tbsp)	0	0.03	0.15	24
Peanuts (1 oz)	0	0.12	0.07	41
Pear (1 medium)	1.60	0.02	0.05	12
Pepper, chile, raw (½ pepper)	21.6	0.03	0.23	10.35
Peppers, sweet (10 strips)	78	0.04	0.13	13
Pie, apple (1 piece)	37	0.03	0.04	32
Pizza, cheese (1 slice)	74	0.20	0.04	35
Pizza, vegetable (1 slice)	58	0.40	0.50	116
Plum (1)	21	0.03	0.05	1.45
Popcorn (1 cup)	0.80	0.02	0.02	2
Pork (3 oz)	0	0.80	0.30	3
Potatoes, mashed (1 cup)	8.40	0.20	0.50	17
Potato salad (1 cup)	2.93	0.20	0.40	19

VITAMIN C (MG)	VITAMIN E (MG)	CALCIUM (MG)	MAGNESIUM (MG)	POTASSIUM (MG)	SELENIUM (MCG)	ZINC (MG)	CALORIES
90/75	15/15	1,000/1,000	420/320	4,700/4,700	55/55	11/8	
0.52	0.12	6	7	22	9	13	41
0.15	0.65	96	15	133	10	0.30	173
6	1.40	41	13	207	11	0.66	216
6	0.70	6	9	186	0.10	0.17	70
0	0	12	51	214	2	1	190
0	2	15	50	186	2	1	165
7	0.20	15	12	198	0.17	0.17	100
65	0.30	6	10	145	0.20	0.12	2
70	0.36	7	6.46	105	0	0	5
4	1.78	13	8	76	1	0.20	296
1	0	117	16	113	13	1	272
79	2	189	65	548	23	2	170
6	0	3	5	114	0.30	0.07	40
0	0	1	11	24	0.80	0.30	31
0	0.20	6	15	253	14	2	191
13	0.04	46	38	621	2	0.60	201
19	0.14	14	36	551	10	0.60	358

(continued)

	VITAMIN A (MCG)	VITAMIN B₁ (THIAMIN) (MG)	VITAMIN B₆ (MG)	FOLATE (MCG)
RDAS FOR MEN/WOMEN	**900/700**	**1.2/1.1**	**1.3/1.3**	**400/400**
Pot pie, chicken	256	0.30	0.20	41
Pretzels (10 twists)	0	0.30	0.07	103
Raisins (1.5 oz)	0	0.05	0.08	1.28
Raspberries (10)	0.38	0.01	0.01	4
Rice, brown (1 cup)	0	0.20	0.30	8
Rice, white (1 cup)	0	0.03	0.15	5
Ricotta cheese, part skim (½ cup)	132	0.03	0.02	16
Salad dressing, light Italian (1 Tbsp)	0	0	0	0
Salmon (3 oz)	9.84	0.20	0.71	22
Salsa (½ cup)	44	0.05	0.16	21
Sauerkraut (1 cup)	1.42	0.03	0.18	34
Sausage (1 link)	0	0.05	0.01	0.26
Shrimp (4 large)	0	0.01	0.03	0.77
Soft drink with caffeine (12 oz)	0	0	0	0
Soup, cream of chicken (1 cup)	179	0.07	0.07	7
Soup, tomato (1 cup)	29.28	0.09	0.11	15

VITAMIN C (MG)	VITAMIN E (MG)	CALCIUM (MG)	MAGNESIUM (MG)	POTASSIUM (MG)	SELENIUM (MCG)	ZINC (MG)	CALORIES
90/75	15/15	1,000/1,000	420/320	4,700/4,700	55/55	11/8	
2	4	33	24	256	0.70	1	484
0	0.21	22	21	88	3	0.50	229
2.30	0.30	12	13	350	0.26	0.08	127
5	0.17	5	4	28	0.04	0.08	10
0	0.06	20	84	84	19	1	216
0	0.06	16	19	55	12	0.80	205
0	0.09	337	19	155	21	1.70	171
0	0	0	0	2	0.20	0	26
0	0.95	11	28	475	35	0.60	175
18	1.53	39	17	275	0.50	0.30	41
21	0.14	43	18	241	0.90	0.30	45
0	0.03	1.30	1.56	25	1.87	0.24	125
0.48	0	9	7	40	9	0.30	22
0	0	10	3	3	0.34	0	154
1.24	0.25	181	17	272	8	0.67	225
66	2	12	7	263	0.50	0.24	180

(continued)

	VITAMIN A (MCG)	VITAMIN B$_1$ (THIAMIN) (MG)	VITAMIN B$_6$ (MG)	FOLATE (MCG)
RDAS FOR MEN/WOMEN	**900/700**	**1.2/1.1**	**1.3/1.3**	**400/400**
Soybeans (1 cup cooked)	14	0.47	0.10	200
Spaghetti with meatballs (1½ cups)	46	0.38	0.43	101
Spareribs (3 oz)	1.91	0.26	0.22	3
Spinach (1 cup)	140	0.02	0.06	58
Steak (different cuts)	0	0.10	0.30	6
Strawberries (1 cup)	1.66	0.03	0.09	40
Submarine sandwich	71	1	0.10	87
Sunflower seeds (¼ cup)	5	0	0.28	82
Sweet potato (1)	350	0.09	0.25	9
Taco salad (1.5 cups)	71	0.10	0.20	83
Toaster pastry (1)	148	0.20	0.20	15
Tofu (4 oz)	4.96	0.10	0.06	19
Tomato (1 medium)	26	0.02	0.05	9
Tuna salad (1 cup)	49	0.06	0.17	16
Turkey, skinless (½ breast)	0	0.16	2.26	31
Vegetable juice (1 cup)	188	0.10	0.30	51

VITAMIN C (MG)	VITAMIN E (MG)	CALCIUM (MG)	MAGNESIUM (MG)	POTASSIUM (MG)	SELENIUM (MCG)	ZINC (MG)	CALORIES
90/75	15/15	1,000/1,000	420/320	4,700/4,700	55/55	11/8	
31	0.02	261	108	970	3	1.64	298
24	4	138	66	718	39	5	545
0	0.20	30	15	204	24	3	338
8	0.60	30	24	167	0.30	0.16	10
0	0.11	4	19	250	12	3.26	217
97	0.50	27	22	253	1	0.20	46
12	0	189	68	394	31	2.60	386
0.50	12	42	127	248	21.42	1.82	205
19	1.42	41	27	348	0.30	0.30	103
4	192	51	416	4	3	0	279
0	0.90	17	12	57	6.30	0.30	204
0	0.01	434	37	150	11	1	75
8	0.33	6	7	146	0	0.11	35
5	2	35	39	365	84	1	383
0	0.30	39	109	1,142	95	5	413
67	12	26	27	467	1	0.50	50

(continued)

	VITAMIN A (MCG)	VITAMIN B₁ (THIAMIN) (MG)	VITAMIN B₆ (MG)	FOLATE (MCG)
RDAS FOR MEN/WOMEN	**900/700**	**1.2/1.1**	**1.3/1.3**	**400/400**
Walnuts (1 cup)	37	0.27	0.70	82
Watermelon (1 wedge)	104	0.20	0.40	6
Wheat germ (½ cup)	0	0.20	0.40	81
Whey protein powder (2 tsp)	0	0	0	0
Wine, red (3.5 oz)	0	0	0.03	2
Wine, white (3.5 oz)	0	0	0.01	0
Yogurt, low-fat (8 oz)	2	0.10	0.09	24

VITAMIN C (MG)	VITAMIN E (MG)	CALCIUM (MG)	MAGNESIUM (MG)	POTASSIUM (MG)	SELENIUM (MCG)	ZINC (MG)	CALORIES
90/75	15/15	1,000/1,000	420/320	4,700/4,700	55/55	11/8	
4	0	73	253	655	21	4.28	654
31	0.40	41	31	479	0.30	0.20	86
0	0	27	275	166	91	14	104
0	0	0	0	260	0	0	21
0	0	8	13	111	0.20	0.10	88
0	0	9	10	80	0.20	0.07	86
1.70	0	415	37	497	11	1.88	193

Conversion Chart

These equivalents have been slightly rounded to make measuring easier.

VOLUME MEASUREMENTS

U.S.	Imperial	Metric
¼ tsp	–	1 ml
½ tsp	–	2 ml
1 tsp	–	5 ml
1 Tbsp	–	15 ml
2 Tbsp (1 oz)	1 fl oz	30 ml
¼ cup (2 oz)	2 fl oz	60 ml
⅓ cup (3 oz)	3 fl oz	80 ml
½ cup (4 oz)	4 fl oz	120 ml
⅔ cup (5 oz)	5 fl oz	160 ml
¾ cup (6 oz)	6 fl oz	180 ml
1 cup (8 oz)	8 fl oz	240 ml

WEIGHT MEASUREMENTS

U.S.	Metric
1 oz	30 g
2 oz	60 g
4 oz (¼ lb)	115 g
5 oz (⅓ lb)	145 g
6 oz	170 g
7 oz	200 g
8 oz (½ lb)	230 g
10 oz	285 g
12 oz (¾ lb)	340 g
14 oz	400 g
16 oz (1 lb)	455 g
2.2 lb	1 kg

LENGTH MEASUREMENTS

U.S.	Metric
¼"	0.6 cm
½"	1.25 cm
1"	2.5 cm
2"	5 cm
4"	11 cm
6"	15 cm
8"	20 cm
10"	25 cm
12" (1')	30 cm

PAN SIZES

U.S.	Metric
8" cake pan	20 × 4 cm sandwich or cake tin
9" cake pan	23 × 3.5 cm sandwich or cake tin
11" × 7" baking pan	28 × 18 cm baking tin
13" × 9" baking pan	32.5 × 23 cm baking tin
15" × 10" baking pan	38 × 25.5 cm baking tin (Swiss roll tin)
1½ qt baking dish	1.5 liter baking dish
2 qt baking dish	2 liter baking dish
2 qt rectangular baking dish	30 × 19 cm baking dish
9" pie plate	22 × 4 or 23 × 4 cm pie plate
7" or 8" springform pan	18 or 20 cm springform or loose-bottom cake tin
9" × 5" loaf pan	23 × 13 cm or 2 lb narrow loaf tin or pâté tin

TEMPERATURES

Fahrenheit	Centigrade	Gas
140°	60°	–
160°	70°	–
180°	80°	–
225°	105°	¼
250°	120°	½
275°	135°	1
300°	150°	2
325°	160°	3
350°	180°	4
375°	190°	5
400°	200°	6
425°	220°	7
450°	230°	8
475°	245°	9
500°	260°	–

Index

Underscored page references indicate boxed text and charts. **Boldface** references indicate illustrations.

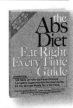